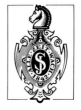

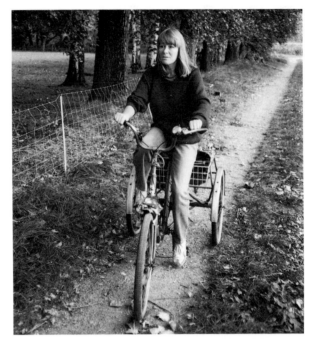

The road was long and hard for Edith but she never gave up.
Six years after onset of right hemiplegia she can at last enjoy
moving and being out of doors again despite her disability.

The road is long
with many a winding turn,
that leads us to who knows where
who knows where . . .

Patricia M. Davies

Right in
the Middle

Selective Trunk Activity in the
Treatment of Adult Hemiplegia

Foreword by Susanne Klein-Vogelbach

With 316 Figures
in 533 Separate Illustrations

Springer-Verlag Berlin Heidelberg New York
London Paris Tokyo Hong Kong

Patricia M. Davies, MCSP Dip. Phys. Ed.
Postgraduate Study Centre, Hermitage
Medical Centre
CH-7310 Bad Ragaz

Written by the same author:

Steps To Follow

A Guide to the Treatment of Adult Hemiplegia

Photographs: David J. Brühwiller and Marianne Tobler, CH-7310 Bad Ragaz
Cover Illustration: Discobolo Lancellotti, Museo Naz. Romano

ISBN 3-540-51242-X Springer-Verlag Berlin Heidelberg New York
ISBN 0-387-51242-X Springer-Verlag New York Berlin Heidelberg

Library of Congress Cataloging-in-Publication Data
Davies, Patricia M. Right in the middle : selective trunk activity in the treatment of adult
hemiplegia / Patricia M. Davies ; foreword by Susanne Klein-Vogelbach. p.   cm.
Includes bibliographical references.
ISBN 0-387-51242-X (U. S.: alk. paper)
1. Hemiplegics - Rehabilitation.   I. Title. [DNLM: 1. Hemiplegia - in adulthood.
2. Hemiplegiarehabilitation. 3.   Physical Therapy.   WL 346 D257r]
RC406.H45D37   1990   616.8'42 - dc20   DNLM/DLC   90-9567

© Springer-Verlag Berlin Heidelberg 1990
Printed in Germany

Typesetting, printing and binding: Appl, Wemding
SPIN: 10476685   21/3130 - 5 4 3 2 – Printed on acid-free paper

Foreword

What is it that characterises Pat Davies' second book about hemiplegia and makes it so special? It is a book which committed therapists can really use in their practical work with patients. We therapists need such books. The engagement and enthusiasm must come from us.

It is similar to a good cookbook. Admittedly one has to know something about cooking but when learning the secrets of haute cuisine – not just the expensive frills but the real refinements – then theoretical dissertations are not very helpful. In practice comments like "you just have to have the right touch" are useless. Many books are disappointing because the reader cannot learn how to put theory into practice, as the author does not disclose the true secrets of his success, perhaps not really wanting the eager students to "bake a good cake" for example.

Such is not the case with this book. In the first theoretical chapter "The Normal Trunk – Evolutionary and Anatomical Considerations" the reader is given information about the significance of the normal anatomical relationships in the development of the body segments: the pelvis, thorax and head. The second chapter, "Aspects of Trunk Control", deals with the muscular control of movement within each of these inherently mobile segments. In the terminology of "Functional Kinetics" the different types of muscle activities are described, defining the importance of the selective use of the musculature in reaction to the pull of gravity. Chapter 3, "Problems Associated with the Loss of Selective Trunk Activity in Hemiplegia" presents Pat Davies' new and important concept for the treatment of patients with hemiplegia, namely, the necessity for regaining selective muscle control of the pelvis, thorax and head. Hence the apt title "Right in the Middle".

The theory is followed by an excellent systematically structured practical section describing activities in lying, in moving between lying and sitting, in sitting, in standing up from sitting, in standing and, before finally the chapter on walking, ball activities to help retrain balance. The determination of a good therapist in action is very much in evidence. The activities have been meticulously and systematically devised and described, giving the reader the feeling of wanting to start working straight away.

The many excellent photographs show the close bond between Pat Davies and her patients. Although the severe disablement caused by the hemiplegia is evident any feeling of hopelessness is driven away by the intensity with which all the patients work with their therapist. The atmosphere is positive and the individual patient's dignity is preserved.

Both fascinating and interesting are the illustrations of young children at different stages of normal motor development, and the way in which the movement patterns shown in them can re-occur later as a result of hermiplegia but are then pathological.

And now a word about the relationship between Pat Davies and myself. We have both gained new insight through working together.

Functional kinetics examines the movement of healthy individuals and tries to find the key to normal movement through the varying intensity of economical activity. The more we succeed in understanding and facilitating movement via perception the clearer the contrast between pathological and normal movement becomes. The concept that every illness is a deficit in health is the approach to treatment using functional kinetics.

As a therapist experienced in the field of neurology Pat Davies travelled from the opposite direction. The wealth of experience with patients taught her to see illness as a lack of health. Through studying pathological manifestations in the periphery she realised the significance of the loss of a sound centre or middle. Functional kinetics starts with a healthy centre and sees disease as an attack on the natural right to be healthy.

Though following two different paths we met somewhere along the way. We were able to learn from one another and never needed to become rivals. This was a gift. It is also a gift for functional kinetics, a concept, which aspires to disclose the secrets of normal movement to all who work in the different specialised fields of physiotherapy.

Bottmingen, March 1990   S. Klein-Vogelbach

Preface

This book is the result of 5 more years of experience with patients who have had the ill fortune to suffer a hemiplegia. It contains recent observations, new ideas and developments in treatment which I believe will lead to a better understanding of the problems and more successful rehabilitation.

After completing my previous book, *Steps to Follow*, I had settled into a state of some complacency. I had many patients to treat, I was the author of a textbook on hemiplegia, and the courses which I was giving were fully booked. The realisation soon dawned, however, that the patients were in no way complacent and kept coming back for more. They longed for more freedom of movement with greater speed and ease and to be able to walk without expending so much energy. They wanted to have the chance to regain some use of their affected hand and not to have to put up with an obviously spastic arm which drew attention to their disability and away from their ability. Their aspirations spurred me on, and I started to write down what I was discovering and doing with my patients, some things with more obvious success than others.

The result was this completely new book, *Right in the Middle*. It does not replace *Steps to Follow* but adds to it and goes further. The activities described in the earlier work for regaining selective activity in the extremities should all be included in the treatment programme, in preparation for functional use. Certain activities, particularly those concerned with retraining balance reactions, have been repeated, but in far more depth and with the emphasis on selective trunk activity: for example, balance reactions in sitting when the weight is shifted sideways.

When using this book and the activities described in it, some important ideas from others should be borne in mind and incorporated into patient assessment and treatment. As the Bobaths have so often said: "The only reply to the question as to whether what you are doing is right for the patient is the reaction of the patient to what you are doing". Certainly spasticity is like a barometer telling the therapist whether the patient is trying too hard, whether the activity is too difficult, or whether she is giving too little support.

Klein-Vogelbach has convincingly taught the importance of exact observation and analysis of movement. She has shown that even the slightest deviation can alter muscle activity completely.

Maitland (1986) advocates checking constantly during a treatment session whether the patient has improved as a result of the therapeutic procedure which has been used. The therapist must select "those subjective and objective findings that must improve if the patient is to be made well again". Movements which are found to be painful or limited during assessment are recorded and then repeated after treatment to note any change in range of movement, in the degree of discomfort or in the pain-range relationship. "Identifying these main assessment markers with a large obvious asterisk not only enforces a commitment but makes retrospective assessments quicker, easier and more complete and therefore more valuable".

When treating a patient with hemiplegia the therapist is well-advised to use a similar system, but with regard to assessing the quality of a certain movement or function which she is presently aiming to improve. Also very much applicable is Maitland's "brick wall concept", a concept in which the X-ray and diagnosis may influence the treatment, but in fact the behaviour of the signs and symptoms guide the therapist. In the treatment of adult hemiplegia a problem-solving approach is used to improve the patient's functional ability and quality of movement by changing the presenting symptoms. Information about the lesion itself only serves to further her knowledge and deepen her understanding.

The patients in the illustrations in this book are at different stages in their rehabilitation. Their hemiplegia was the result of stroke, aneurysm, tumour or head injury. The patients' ages range from 15–75 years, but age really does not make that much difference to rehabilitation (Adler et al. 1980). The terms "sound side", "hemiplegic side" and "affected side" have been used for clarity when describing the assessment and treatment, but it should not be forgotten that the sides of the body are dependent upon one another for normal movement. The lesion is a central one and will as such influence both sides to some degree (Brodal 1973).

In the text the patient is referred to as "he" and the therapist as "she". In the figure legends, the correct personal pronoun has been used. Some of the patients have a left hemiplegia and others a right, and the side of the paralysis is clearly indicated.

The book is meant to be used in clinical practice; the activities should be tried out, built on and improved. Treatment should never become static but continue to develop further and further according to the needs of the patients.

During treatment every effort should be made to achieve the so-called "flow state" for the patient, a state described by Csikszentmihalyi in which "the individual steps beyond the apparent limitations of the self" (*Newsweek,* 2 June 1986). Such a flow state exists when the task at hand and the individual's skill are equally matched. Challenges that are greater than the skills cause anxiety, and if the skills exceed the challenge, then boredom is the result. When the skill meets the challenge, the therapy sessions will be more stimulating, enjoyable and productive and the patient will be spared the indignity of being labelled as "unmotivated".

The Barthel Index (Mahoney and Barthel 1965) is probably the most widely used scale for evaluating activities of daily living for research purposes (Wade and Langton Hewer 1987). However useful it may be in the assessment of a patient's ability to perform basic self-care tasks independently, it should never be used as a basis for discontinuing treatment, as has been suggested. There is certainly more to life than a 100% Barthel Index rating!

With the treatment described in this book the patient's ability should continue to improve over a long period of time. Whenever possible such treatment should be available for the patient for as long as it continues to improve his quality of life, and certainly until he can move about freely outside the confines of his home.

Bad Ragaz, April 1990   Pat Davies

Acknowledgements

This book would never have been written had I not been privileged to meet and learn from Karel and Bertie Bobath. Their concept has been the basis of my work and its development for the past 20 years. I would like to thank them for their enormous contribution to patients with hemiplegia all over the world and to us, the therapists who treat them.

I should also like to thank the members of the International Association of Bobath Instructors (IBITAH) for their very positive response when I first presented my work on selective trunk activity to them at the 3rd International meeting back in 1987. Their enthusiastic reception encouraged me to complete the book, and the exchange of ideas made possible through the association has been a constant stimulation.

I am most grateful to Susanne Klein-Vogelbach for enabling me to take a new look at the trunk and giving me an insight into the intricacies of the abdominal muscles and their function. Many of the activities described in this book are based on her unique ideas and I am honoured that she agreed to write the foreword.

I am indebted to Jürg Kesselring for correcting the manuscript and for inspiring me to keep at it until the job was done. My thanks go as well to his wonderful secretary, Anni Guntli, who transformed my chaotic hand-written pages into an orderly manuscript, and to Evi Nigg who also helped by typing some of the earlier chapters in her free time.

My thanks go to Herta Göller for giving up her holiday time to discuss ideas with me, to file the masses of references and above all for undertaking the mammoth task of translating the book into German.

My thanks also to Urban Diethelm, who shared books and references with me and provided X-rays for the illustrations, and to Marianne Brune who spent a week-end sorting the many photographs into numerical order.

I should like to thank the parents of the delightful babies for taking time to come to the studio and making the comparative illustrations possible.

My very special thanks go to all the patients who never gave up and so encouraged me to go on searching for new answers, I should particularly like to thank those patients and their partners who were always so willing to spend hours in the studio to make the illustrations possible. Without their help the book would have been a dull dissertation indeed, lacking the clarity which the photographs provide.

I should like to express my gratitude to all members of the staff of Springer-Verlag who helped, encouraged and made my job easier right to the end of what proved to be a long time, and for such insightful editing and production. A special thank you must certainly go to Bernhard Lewerich for all his guidance and inspiration, and to Marga Botsch his assistant who lightened my load in so many ways.

I am deeply indebted to my friend and partner, Gisela Rolf, who supported me unstintingly during the long writing process. She was always ready to share ideas, make helpful suggestions, give positive criticism and take care of myriad unseen chores so that I could have time to sit down and write.

Contents

Introduction

The importance of selective trunk activity in the rehabilitation of the hemiplegic patient, has, I believe, been grossly underestimated. The loss, often total, of such selective activity has not even been fully realised. Reading through recent literature on the subject of hemiplegia, I found only scant reference to the trunk muscles in a very small percentage of them, and nothing at all about their selective activity.

A computer search through the Washington Library of Congress revealed that over 5000 articles had been published on the subject of hemiplegia during the last 20 years. The computer showed a stubbornly repeated zero, however, when the word hemiplegia was coupled with abdominal muscles, trunk muscles, trunk activity etc.

There were many articles on the recovery of motor function, but only referring to upper and lower limb muscles. There were many describing shoulder pain, slings and splints and also walking aids, but even those referring to gait made no reference to the muscles of the trunk. In the work done by Badke and Duncan (1983) on the patterns of rapid motor responses during postural adjustments when standing, only the activity in the muscles of the ankle, knee and hip were examined. The same applied to the study done by Hockermann et al. (1984) on platform training and postural stability in hemiplegia, even though it could well have been that the improvement which was noted in the patients who had been trained on the moving platform stemmed from increased activity in the muscles of the trunk.

It is hard to understand why the trunk has been so neglected, not only in the literature, but also in the different rehabilitation approaches. The biggest part of the body, the centre piece, in fact, has somehow been all but ignored. I, too, in the past have failed to observe and understand the problems in this essential area during 25 years of working almost exclusively with patients who had suffered neurological lesions. During 8 years working in the field of traumatic tetra- and paraplegia, my first job being at the National Centre for Spinal Cord Injuries, Stoke Mandeville, UK, the significance of the trunk muscles, in particular the abdominal muscles, was clear to all of us then, but the problem resulting from a spinal cord lesion was far simpler.

According to the level of the lesion, the patient either had abdominal muscle activity or he did not, and the extensor muscles with their segmental innervation were paralysed below approximately the same level as the abdominals were. We, as physiotherapists, learned to assist the patient when he could not cough unaided, and we diligently strengthened the latissimus dorsi as a substitute for other trunk muscles, following the convincing teaching of Sir Ludwig Guttmann. The methods used have been comprehensively described in the well-illustrated books by Bromley (1976) and Rolf et al. (1973).

The problems caused by the absent trunk activity were not difficult to understand because there was a balance between the flexor and extensor paralysis. There was also a certain reflex tone in the muscles due to reflex activity at a spinal level, and even the loss of sensation had a level which was clearly demarcated.

During subsequent years I became increasingly fascinated by the problems confronting patients who had suffered a lesion of the brain and set out to further my knowledge and my treatment skills. For the past 20 years I have been involved in this task, treating patients with every form of upper motor neurone lesion, particularly those with cerebral lesions, and searching for a way to improve treatment. I often wonder now how, during all those years of working with neurologically involved patients, despite careful assessment and analysis of their movements, I took so long to see that a key problem was the loss of selective trunk activity.

It was not that I had ignored the trunk as such. I spent 6 months studying proprioceptive neuromuscular facilitation techniques (PNF) in Vallejo, California, USA, with Margaret Knott, which entailed many hours of practising patterns for strengthening the trunk muscles, including a specific emphasis on m. quadratus lumborum. The PNF patterns, however, were mass patterns of trunk activity (Knott and Voss 1960) either for the flexors or extensors, but not selective, and usually combined with the same activity in the legs, the arms or the neck.

Shortly afterwards I attended a course on the neurodevelopmental treatment of cerebral palsied children at the Bobath Centre in London and at the end of the 2 months started working with Karel and Bertha Bobath at their centre. In the Bobath concept, the trunk and its rotation is stressed as a key to reducing hypertonicity, moving proximally to inhibit distal spasticity.

Later at King's College Hospital, London, and then for the following 12 years in Switzerland I continued to treat patients with upper motor neurone lesions, particularly those with hemiplegia. At last, about 5 years ago I realised why my patients had not been able to achieve greater freedom of movement. I had not given selective trunk activity the same meticulous attention and training which I had given to the selective activity of the upper and lower extremities. It was not a sudden realisation. It gradually dawned on me through a series of events and the exchange of ideas with other therapists. Through my interest in patients with the pusher syndrome (Davies 1985), I had observed the loss of muscle tone and activity in the abdominal muscles on the affected side of the body and the effect which this loss had on movement and balance.

My patients are required to undress adequately for treatment and wear bathing suits or gymnastic shorts, and I became more and more aware of the position of their navels and how these moved when the patients moved. As a result I started to study my own navel and found I knew very little about its normal behaviour as a point of reference during the activities of daily life. Joan Mohr came from the United States of America to give advanced courses on the treatment of adult hemiplegia (Bobath concept) in Bad Ragaz. As her organising assistant I was able to watch her working with patients, using different ways to activate the muscles of the trunk, including balancing on a moving ball. My interest was aroused, but I was not completely satisfied because there was too little selective activity in the trunk itself and between the limbs and the trunk. Perhaps the major contribution Joan Mohr made to my learning process was her description of the development of trunk activity in normal babies, with extensor control preceding flexor control, and how the eventual rotation is dependent upon both of these (Mohr 1984, 1985, 1987).

The final enlightenment dawned during the years in which I came to know Dr. Susanne Klein-Vogelbach and her work. Susanne Klein-Vogelbach, a brilliant physiotherapist, had already in 1963 delivered a lecture in Munich, which was published in the same year, on the stabilisation of the centre of the body and the necessary adaptive buttressing mechanisms as being the starting point for the re-education of movement, with particular reference to the problems of hemiplegia (Klein-Vogelbach 1963). Since 1977 I have continued to learn from her through personal discussions, attending a 4-week course, studying her books, listening to her lecturing and, perhaps most of all, through watching her work with some of my patients.

Through my continued work with patients with hemiplegia I had also come to realise that the loss of selective trunk activity was also a loss of the ability to isolate the activity in the limbs from that in the trunk. The patient is unable, for example, to extend his hips when the lower trunk requires flexor activity or to extend the lower trunk when the hips are flexed. In addition, I began to understand that the abdominal muscles could only work optimally if the thorax could be stabilised adequately, and that these muscles provided the fundamental basis for almost all normal economical movements.

Despite its obvious importance, the trunk has, however, been relatively neglected in the various rehabilitation programmes. The following possibilities could explain why regaining selective trunk activity has been emphasised so little in the treatment of the hemiplegic patient, and why the loss of abdominal muscle tone and activity has not been observed:

1. The majority of therapists fail to undress their patients adequately for treatment and have therefore not noticed the loss of muscle activity and the resulting alternative movements which the patient uses to compensate for the loss. In the numerous hospitals and rehabilitation centres which I have visited, the patient is usually wearing a tracksuit while being treated, or often his normal clothing, with perhaps the leg of the trousers rolled up to expose the knee. He often wears a shirt or even a pullover so that the muscles of the trunk, especially the anterior ones, cannot be seen at all, particularly as the patient is usually sitting or standing in a kyphotic position, with the clothing folding loosely over his chest and abdomen.

2. The possibilities for compensatory or alternative movements are numerous because of the many joints which are involved and also because of the extremely complex musculature in the area. A minimal shift of weight, perhaps less than a centimetre sideways, forwards or backwards can change the muscle activity from flexor to extensor or even to the hip muscles.

3. The activity of the abdominal muscles is manifold and so discreet at times that it cannot be directly observed when compared with the obvious functioning of muscles such as the elbow flexors or the knee extensors when these act to move or to prevent movement of more distal parts of the body. Therapists and the rehabilitation team as a whole, therefore, do not fully understand the subtle workings of the abdominal muscles. Instead, they concentrate on the mechanically simpler limb-moving muscles which can more easily be observed in action.

   Unlike most other muscles in the body, the abdominals can shorten or lengthen selectively in part and not only as a whole. In their role as stabilisers they are constantly adapting, and these changes in length or tension cannot be directly seen.

4. The literature is limited and apart from providing anatomical descriptions of the various muscles of the trunk is of little help to the therapist. Even in such classical textbooks as *Gray's Anatomy,* the explanation of the action of the abdominal muscles is oversimplified and nonspecific (Williams and Warwick 1980).

5. For more than 40 years the Bobaths have been teaching the importance of inhibiting spasticity or hypertonicity as being the key to regaining normal movement patterns in hemiplegia. As a result, although Bertha Bobath herself stresses the need to assess each patient individually, as flaccidity may be an additional problem, many therapists are so conditioned that they see the affected trunk side in all hemiplegics as being shortened by the pull of spastic muscles. In most cases, however, careful examination will reveal that the lower trunk side is in fact too long, i. e. hypotonic. The apparent shortening of the trunk on the hemiplegic side is usually due to one of the following:

   - The elevators of the shoulder girdle are inactive with perhaps too little tone, and the shoulder hangs down.
   - The depressors of the scapula are spastic and the shoulder girdle is pulled downwards as a result.
   - When moving in sitting or in standing the patient elevates his sound shoulder vigorously in his efforts to maintain the upright position against gravity, and the contralateral side of his trunk shortens as a result.
   - The patient is unable to or afraid of taking weight through the affected leg. He stands with his weight shifted over the sound side and the opposite side of his trunk shortens to maintain balance.
   - Loss of selective extensor activity in the affected leg causes the foot to plantarflex during weight bearing. The plantar flexion of the foot against the floor pushes the pelvis upwards on that side.
   - During the stance phase of walking, the abductors of the affected hip fail

to control the lateral shift of the pelvis. The hip adducts and the hemiplegic side shortens reactively.
- To take a step forwards with the hemiplegic leg, the patient uses active flexion of the whole limb in a mass synergy. The pelvis is lifted up, elevation being part of the total flexor pattern of the lower limb.

Whatever the reasons for the relative neglect of the trunk may have been, it is important that the retraining and regaining of selective trunk activity, and trunk activity independent from the activity taking place in the limbs, should be an integral part of the rehabilitation programme for patients with hemiplegia. Since integrating the activities and ideas which are presented in this book in the treatment programme for my patients, I have been amazed by the results. Patients who have for years been dependent upon a stick to maintain their balance while walking, have voluntarily discarded the support after a relatively short period of intensive treatment. They are no longer afraid to walk freely, as they perceive the increased stability which they have acquired. Other patients have become able to walk at a more normal speed, far faster than before, to the great relief of their relatives. Some patients who after months or even years of previous treatment could only move their arm in primitive mass movement synergies have regained the ability to bring their hand forward to perform tasks.

When teaching selective trunk activity the following points deserve particular consideration:

1. Attention to details. Essential for successful treatment is the exactness with which the activities are carried out. As I have already mentioned, the possibility for alternative evasive movements is great, and it is incumbent upon the therapist to enable the patient to perform the movement correctly. The harder the patient tries to move on his own, the more he will be forced to use compensatory mechanisms. In his eagerness to follow the instructions of the therapist and succeed, he reinforces the movement by overactivating the sound side or by using the developmentally earlier extensor muscles of the trunk. The guiding principle for the correct performance of the activities is that the therapist should demand less of the patient and by so doing achieve more.

2. Moving without over-exertion. "The key to learning something new is often in preventing unwanted responses, which leads to the discovery of appropriate effort" (Gelb 1987). The paradox "give up trying too hard, but never give up" which Gelb describes as being the heart of the Alexander Technique, is a very good maxim for both the patient and his therapist.
     The therapist's hands should support the patient in such a way that he is able to move without over-exertion.

3. Normalising tone. Following the principles of the Bobath concept, tone must be normalised before an active movement is facilitated. If hypertonus is present, the therapist first inhibits spasticity until no resistance is felt when she moves the patient's body or part of it in the desired movement sequence. Tone should be carefully increased if it is too low as the patient will otherwise use effort or compensatory mechanisms to perform the required activity, e. g. he will raise his shoulders and extend his neck when standing up from sitting to compensate for insufficient active extension in his lower limb. Distal hypertonus will often be increased as a result.

4. Verbal communication. By moving the patient with her hands in the way she wants him to move, and then asking him to perform the movement with her, the therapist can avoid using long confusing verbal instructions. Her verbal commands are reduced to a minimum, and her voice should be used in such a way that the patient moves without effort in an economical, harmonious manner. The actual words which the therapist uses can also effect the quality of the movement, and reduce the amount of over-activity from alternative muscles. By changing the way in which she asks for activity she can markedly influence the reaction of the patient. For example, the therapist wishes the seated patient to keep his arm forwards with his hand against her hand and his elbow extended. If she uses the command "push against my hand", the patient will lean forward from the hips and use his back and neck extensors strongly in his attempt to perform the required exercise. By placing the patient's hand against her hand, in the desired position and merely saying quietly, "just stay here, shoulder forward", the quality of the stabilisation of the trunk by the abdominals and the activity in the elbow extensors will immediately be improved.

5. Weight control. It is most important that the patient does not gain excessive weight, and if overweight is already a problem, he should be helped and encouraged to reduce. Caix et al. (1984) found a distinct correlation between obesity and abdominal muscle activity in normal subjects: "It was also seen that the capacities of the abdominal wall of obese subjects were greatly reduced regarding tonus and posture and were practically nil with respect to movement" (Caix et al. 1984). Obesity can also cause raised blood pressure and increase the risk of second stroke (Truswell 1986). Cosmetically, the patient will enjoy both his improved appearance and being able to wear fashionable clothes again after he has lost weight or if he maintains his correct weight.

Improved function of the upper limbs, improved quality of walking and confident balance during all activities and in all situations can only be achieved by improving selective trunk activity, particularly that of the abdominal muscles. I believe the key to successful treatment lies in the regaining of adaptive stabilisation of the trunk and the ability to move parts of it in isolation.

Part I
Theoretical Antecedents

1 The Normal Trunk
– Evolutionary and Anatomical Considerations

Since human beings adopted the upright posture and began to walk on two legs instead of four, an elaborate extensor musculature has been required to hold the body erect against gravity. The vertebral column became exposed to new patterns of force through the different weight distribution and muscle tension. Because of the very much narrower base provided by only two legs, an intricate system of balance reactions became necessary, and the trunk naturally formed the foundation for such a mechanism.

The hands, freed from their weight-bearing and balancing tasks, became more and more skilled in their activity, and the trunk had to provide a mobile, yet stable support to bring them into – and hold them in – every conceivable position for their skilled actions.

To lighten the work of the trunk for biped stance and walking, the lower vertebrae fused to form the pillar of the sacrum, inserted like a wedge between the two sides of the pelvis, with the four rudimentary vertebrae fused to form a small triangular bone below it.

The sacrum is joined to the pelvis, a bony girdle massively constructed to withstand compression and the stresses of dynamic body weight and powerful musculature (Fig. 1.1). The sacro-iliac joint with its very restricted movements is inherently strong and further stabilised by massive ligaments. Together, these

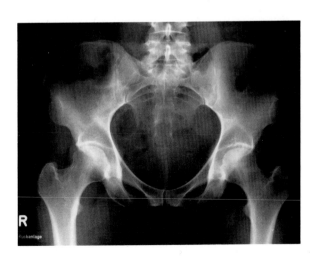

Fig. 1.1. X-ray of normal pelvis. The massive construction of the pelvis withstands compression and provides a stable origin for powerful muscles

intrinsically stable structures are primarily concerned with transmitting the weight of the head, trunk and arms above to the legs below. The pelvis also provides surfaces for the attachment of powerful muscles of the trunk and lower limbs.

The pelvic girdle, as a whole, forms a stable base for the long moving lever of the trunk in upright postures. The connection between the trunk and the upper limbs is quite different as the scapula "floats in a muscular suspension" (Williams and Warwick 1980) (Fig. 1.2) in order to allow a great range of movement possibilities for the grasping hand.

The scapulae are very closely related to the hands and make it possible for them to explore and experience the environment from early childhood onwards. As Middendorf (1987) writes, it is as if "our shoulder blades are our interior hands, and in appearance are anatomically similar to the exterior hands with regard to shape and size" (Fig. 1.3). To allow for a freer range of movement at the shoulder, the scapula orientation changed, so that the glenoid fossa faces more laterally.

With this reorganisation of the shoulder came a change in the shape of the thorax as well, so that its maximum diameter is now transverse, and not dorsoventral as in quadrupeds. The shoulder girdle, unlike the plevic girdle, has no direct articulation with the vertebral column and is therefore dependant on complex muscle activity to provide the necessary support for the moving arm (Fig. 1.4).

Gray's Anatomy gives a clearly depicted comparison between the two bony girdles:

Pectoral girdle	*Pelvic girdle*
1. Dermal and endochondral	Entirely endochondral
2. Two components, clavicle and scapula, which remain separate	Three components, pubis, ischium and ilium, which fuse into a single innominate bone

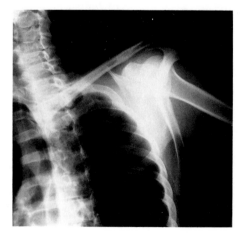

Fig. 1.2. X-ray of normal shoulder girdle. The freely moving scapula enables the hand to be brought into countless positions for performing skilled tasks

3. No articulation with vertebral column	Articulates with the sacral vertebrae
4. No direct ventral articulation (clavicles connected only by intraclavicular ligament)	Direct ventral articulation at symphysis pubis
5. Articulations of clavicles with axial skeleton (sternum) are relatively small, mobile and ventral	Articulations of innominate bones with axial skeleton (sacrum) are relatively large, capable of little movement, and dorsal
6. Comparatively lightly built for mobility	Massively constructed for resistance to stress rather than for mobility
7. Resilient to thrust	Transmits thrust between vertebral column and leg
8. Shallow joint with limb, allowing wide range of movement	Deep joint with limb, limiting range of movement

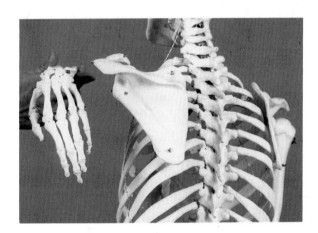

Fig. 1.3. The hand and the scapula are anatomically similar in both shape and size

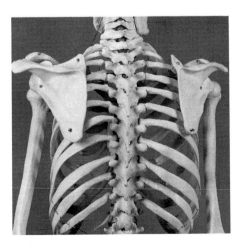

Fig. 1.4. The shoulder girdle is not directly connected to the vertebral column. Complex muscle activity supports the moving arm

Between the shoulder girdle and the pelvic girdle is the long flexible lever of the trunk. It is clear that without a stable supporting central point, the muscles of the upper limbs would have no anchorage. The same applies in the case of the lower limbs as soon as one foot is lifted from the floor and the pelvis becomes dependent upon the stabilisation from above. Likewise the weight of the head could not be supported against gravity during movement as the muscles of the neck are also attached to the upper trunk.

1.1 The Vertebral Column

The enormous variety of movements of the trunk is made possible by the construction of the vertebral column, consisting of a series of short levers joined together. The bodies of the movable vertebrae are strongly bound to each other by the fibrocartilagenous intervertebral discs and together form a continuous flexible pillar which supports the weight of the head, the arms and the trunk. The mechanical arrangement ist unstable and dependent upon intricate muscle activity to control the movements of the individual joints in relation to one another.

1.1.1 Movements of the Vertebral Column

The range of movement possible between two adjoining vertebrae is relatively small, restricted by the limited amount of change which can occur in the shape of the intervertebral disc and by the shape of the articular facets of the vertebrae themselves. The spinal column when considered as a whole entity, however, has a considerable range of movement due to the summation of these small movements throughout its length.

The spine can flex forwards, extend backwards, flex sideways or rotate, but as Grieve (1981) states: "Pure movement in one plane perhaps does not exist". Although there is considerable individual variation in the amount of segmental movement possible, he depicts average ranges gathered from a variety of sources (Figs. 1.5, 1.6). The movement possibilities in the thoracic spine are seen to be more limited than in the other areas, thus reducing interference with respiration to a minimum. The limitation is not only due to the shape of the joints between the vertebrae themselves, but also to the restriction caused by the rib cage.

Axial rotation is, however, surprisingly free despite the rib attachments and normally ranges between 60°–80° to each side (Dvorak and Dvorak 1983), which exceeds to amount of rotation possible in the lumbar spine by far. Such freedom of rotation in the thoracic spine is necessary if the hands are to be brought into appropriate positions for functional tasks.

Clinically, when the spine is fully extended, rotation in both the upper and lower thoracic areas feels blocked. The clinical feeling that rotation is very

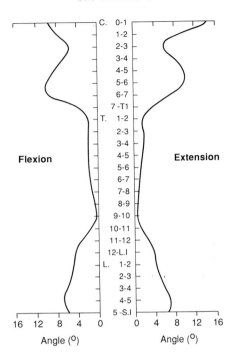

Fig. 1.5. Average ranges of segmental movement within the vertebral column: flexion and extension. (From Grieve 1981)

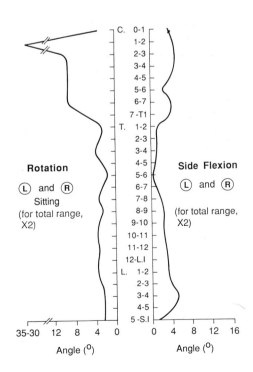

Fig. 1.6. Average ranges of segmental movement within the vertebral column: rotation and side flexion. (From Grieve 1981). Freedom of rotation in the thoracic spine allows the hands to be moved into functional positions to either side of the midline

much limited by extension is supported by Grieve (1986) when describing the testing of the combined movements, extension with right side flexion and right side rotation: "This combination creates a severe 'jamming' effect on the facet joints in conjunction with a reduction in size of the intervertebral foramen". He also writes that: "Accompanying rotation, the upper vertebra of a motion segment will tend to tilt forwards (flexion)".

Certainly at the level of the thoraco-lumbar mortise joint extension prevents rotation altogether. "The transition from thoracic to lumbar characteristics may occur at segments T10–T11 or T11–T12 or T12–L1. The transition is most marked by a singular configuration of articular processes of one vertebra which has the effect of forming with the subjacent vertebra a mortise and tenon joint when under compression or extension; this is one of the very few examples of complete bone-to-bone 'lock' in the body. On extension, the lower facets of the transitional vertebra lock into the upper facets of the uppermost 'lumbar-type' vertebra, and no movement other than flexion is then possible". (Grieve 1981 p. 14).

Rotation in the lumbar spine is also limited in extension by contact of the facet joint planes which Grieve describes as being like "the flanges on train-wheels".

1.1.2 Movements of the Rib Cage

The individual ribs have their own range and direction of movement, and these combine to enable the characteristic respiratory excursions of the thorax. Each rib can be regarded as a lever, with its fulcrum adjacent to its costo-transverse joint. As the shaft of the rib elevates, the neck depresses, or vice versa. Because there is such a big difference in the length of the two arms of the lever, a small movement at the vertebral end causes a far greater movement at the anterior extremity of the rib. The head of each rib articulates with the body of the vertebra, and only a slight gliding movement is possible between the articular surfaces because of the fixation of the ligaments. In the same way, strong ligaments bind the necks and tubercles of the ribs to the transverse processes of the vertebrae, allowing only a slight gliding movement at the costo-transverse joints as well. The joints of the heads of the ribs and the costo-transverse joints move simultaneously and in the same direction so that the neck of the rib moves as if on a single joint.

It is clear, therefore, that when the thoracic spine is extended, the necks of the ribs are depressed and the long lever effect magnifies the elevation of the anterior rib cage. During normal inspiration, however, extension of the thoracic spine is automatically counteracted by appropriate muscle tension anteriorly, and conversely during expiration, the extensors of the spine prevent a flexion movement.

When the third to the sixth ribs elevate, their anterior extremities carry the body of the sternum forwards and upwards. The costal cartilages of the vertebrochondral ribs, including the seventh rib, articulate with one another and

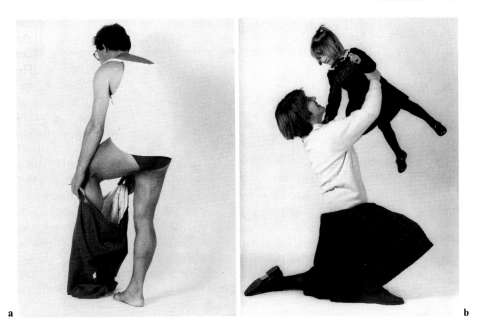

Fig. 1.7 a, b. The trunk provides a stable, yet dynamic foundation for all movement. **a** Ease and independence in daily life activities. **b** Fulfillment of individual wishes

each pushes the one above it upwards till finally the lower end of the body of the sternum is pushed forwards and upwards.

1.2 Conclusion

Despite the need for the trunk to be held upright and stable against gravity, it also needs to be freely movable so that it can be brought into the innumerable positions required for the countless activities each person takes so much for granted to fulfill the needs and wishes of his daily life (Fig. 1.7 a, b). Posture has been succinctly described as being "arrested movement" at any moment during activity (K. Bobath 1980) which perhaps conveys the enormous variety of possible positions for the trunk and the extremities.

As Samson Wright (1945) points out "it must be emphasized that posture is the basis of movement, and all movements start and finish in posture". Every movement which is made, and each posture which is held requires that muscles act in order to exert control against the pull of gravity – either to move against the pull, to control the speed of the movement in the direction of the pull or to prevent any movement despite the pull.

2 Aspects of Trunk Control

If the vertebral column is considered as a series of small levers, each vertebra moving in relation to the adjacent ones as well as together with them, it becomes obvious that very finely co-ordinated muscle activity is necessary to move or stabilise the spine. Likening the vertebrae to a set of toy building blocks, it would be possible to position such blocks one upon the other so that they would stand precariously balanced. The slightest movement of one of the blocks, or the surface on which the lowest stands, however, would cause them to fall to the ground.

In humans the ideal of absolute balance is only closely approached – and then only momentarily – but never completely reached. Steindler (1955) showed that a completely passive equilibrium is impossible because the centres of gravity of the links of the spinal column and the movement centres of the joints between them cannot all be brought to coincide perfectly with the common line of gravity. A patient with a complete spinal cord lesion below C4 or C5 can be carefully positioned in sitting until the therapist is able to remove her hands, and he remains balanced and upright. The patient needs only to alter the position of his head or lift one arm forwards, and he, too, would fall over as the paralysed muscles could not make the necessary adjustment. In a position of relaxed standing or sitting, we, too, can find a position in which our muscle activity is reduced to a minimum, the shape of the vertebrae and their supporting ligaments reducing the need for muscular control. The moment the body is moved out of the line of gravity, however, muscular activity is called for to bring it back into line or to hold it in the new position. Murray et al. (1975) found a large area of stability over which weight can be shifted and maintained by normal subjects.

All movements of the spine require muscle activity to oppose the pull of gravity. The moment the body moves behind, forwards or sideways from the centre of gravity, the muscles have to act. It is often misunderstood which muscles must be activated to prevent falling or the tendency to fall in a certain direction. For the therapist it is most important that she understands the mechanism clearly as the activities used to activate the trunk muscles selectively will often involve moving the patient in such a way in relation to the pull of gravity, that activity in the desired muscles is stimulated. The ideas presented by Klein-Vogelbach (1990) of a "bridge" and a "tentacle" help to clarify the analysis of the muscle activity.

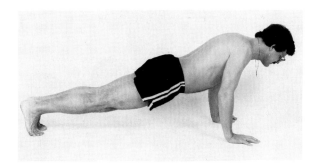

Fig. 2.1. Performing a push-up. The arch of the bridge is supported by the muscles on its underside (normal model)

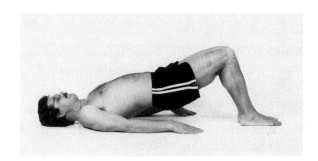

Fig. 2.2. "Bridging". The back and hip extensors support the arch of the bridge (normal model)

2.1 The Bridge

A "bridge" is formed when two parts of the body, in contact with a supporting surface, hold that part of the body situated between them away from the supporting surface. The arch of such a bridge is maintained by the muscles on the underside of the arch being activated.

Example 1. When performing push-ups the arms and the legs form the pillars of the bridge, and the trunk and hips the arch of the bridge (Fig. 2.1). The muscles which support the arch are those on its underside in this case the abdominals and hip flexors, while the lower back extensors remain relaxed (Pauly and Steele 1966).

Example 2. When a person lies on his back with his hips and knees bent and raises his buttocks off the supporting surface ("bridging"), the back and hip extensors support the arch of the bridge (Fig. 2.2).

2.2 The Tentacle

A "tentacle" is a part of the body which moves against the pull of gravity with its distal extremity free, in the sense of not being supported. If the part is not

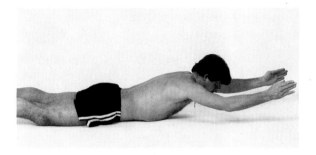

Fig. 2.3. Prone lying, lifting the head and shoulders off the floor. The "tentacle" is supported by the muscles on its uppermost side (normal model)

absolutely vertical, the muscle activity to support the "tentacle" will take place in those muscle groups on its uppermost side in relation to the pull of gravity.

Example 1. Prone lying, lifting the head and shoulders from the supporting surface without using the arms. The muscles holding the "tentacle" are the back and neck extensors (Fig. 2.3).

Example 2. Sitting with the feet remaining on the floor, and leaning backwards. The "tentacle" here is formed by the trunk and head, and the muscles supporting it are those on the uppermost side, namely, the anterior muscles of the neck, the abdominals and hip flexors (Fig. 2.4a, b). Conversely, the moment the trunk is brought forwards in relation to the line of gravity, the extensors of the neck and back spring into action (Fig. 2.4c).

Likewise, in standing, when the body is displaced backwards or forwards, the muscles on the uppermost side of both legs and trunk, in relation to the pull of gravity, will be activated. Brooks (1986) describes activity in the paraspinals, hamstrings and gastrocnemius during forward sway caused by movement of a supporting platform, and activity in the abdominals, rectus femoris, belly of quadriceps and anterior tibialis during backward sway. The whole length of the body forms the "tentacle" in this example.

2.3 The Bridge-Tentacle

The bridge and the tentacle are combined in certain movements, and the muscle activity changes accordingly as the muscles on the uppermost side of the bridge will need to be activated as well in order to anchor the tentacle arising from it. For example, during the activity of "bridging", with the buttocks lifted off the supporting surface, the arch of the bridge is maintained by the muscles on its underside. If, however, one foot is raised in the air, the whole leg becomes a tentacle and the muscles on the uppermost side of the arch are activated as well to support the tentacle, in this case the oblique abdominal muscles (Fig. 2.5a). If one of the arms is lifted, too, the activity increases still further (Fig. 2.5b).

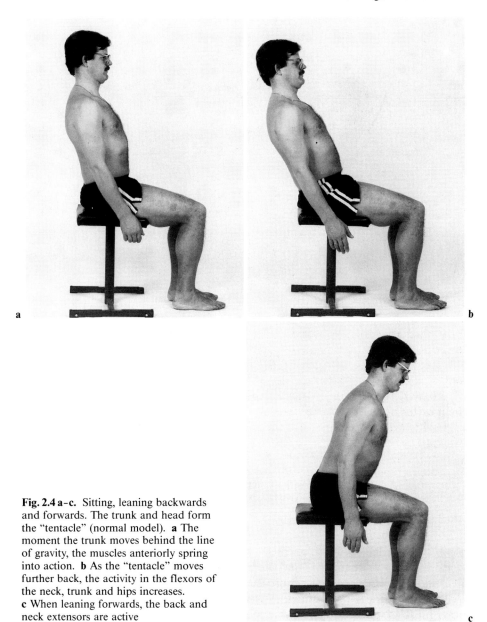

Fig. 2.4 a–c. Sitting, leaning backwards and forwards. The trunk and head form the "tentacle" (normal model). **a** The moment the trunk moves behind the line of gravity, the muscles anteriorly spring into action. **b** As the "tentacle" moves further back, the activity in the flexors of the neck, trunk and hips increases. **c** When leaning forwards, the back and neck extensors are active

2.3.1 Muscular Control of the Trunk

The trunk can move by flexing, extending, side flexing and rotating, or two or more of these may be combined in movement or posture. The principles apply-ing to the "bridge" and the "tentacle" continue to hold true.

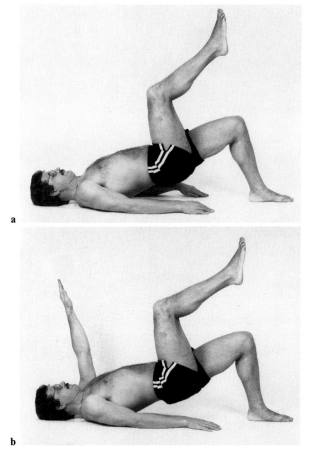

Fig. 2.5 a, b. "Bridging" with one foot lifted off the floor (normal model). **a** The muscles on the uppermost side of the bridge work to support the "bridge-tentacle". **b** Raising the arm as well increases abdominal muscle activity

The two groups of muscles chiefly responsible for moving or controlling the trunk are the back extensors and the muscles which form the abdominal wall. Because of their mechanical arrangement and perhaps their multiple segmental innervation, the abdominal muscles have a peculiar property. They, unlike most other muscles in the body, are able to contract in part and not just as a whole (Platzer 1984; Spaltenholz 1901), making possible the enormous variety of trunk movements and postures and providing a stable anchorage for the muscles which act on the head, shoulder and hip.

As Bobath (1971) explains, the normal postural reflex mechanism requires many and varied degrees of reciprocal innervation. "This is necessary both for the postural fixation of the proximal parts of the body and the regulation of the smooth interaction of the muscles of the moving distal parts".

2.3.2 Anatomical Considerations

Detailed descriptions of the individual muscles of the trunk are to be found in the many anatomy textbooks available. The same applies to those muscles which connect the limbs to the trunk, and are dependent upon it for their efficient action. It is, however, important for the therapist to study the illustrations presented in this chapter and to consider various muscle relationships.

2.3.2.1 Extension

The muscles which extend the trunk against gravity are large and powerful, as they need to be to support the weight of the head and the long levers formed by the arms during functional activities (Fig. 2.6 a). Many of them have attachments to the ribs. Thus, directly, or indirectly through extending the spine, almost all will depress the necks of the ribs posteriorly, causing elevation of their shafts anteriorly (Fig. 2.6 b, c). The elevation of the rib cage anteriorly is greatly magnified because of the large difference in the length of the arms of the lever formed by each rib. A slight movement at the vertebral end of the rib will cause a far greater movement at its anterior extremity. Conversely, if the ribs are elevated anteriorly, as during inspiratory movements of the rib cage, then the spine tends to extend. Both the elevation of the rib cage due to extension of the spine and the extension of the thoracic spine secondary to rib elevation are counteracted by the adaptive activity in the abdominal muscles.

2.3.2.2 Shoulder Girdle

Because the shoulder girdle has no dirrect articulation with the vertebral column, it is very much dependent upon complex muscular activity in order to provide a stable, yet fully dynamic foundation for the moving arm. "The serratus anterior which together with the pectoralis minor, draws the scapula forwards, is the chief muscle concerned in all reaching and pushing movements" (Gray 1980). It also plays an important part in both upward and downward rotation of the scapula.

Both serratus anterior and the pectoralis minor insert on to the rib cage and are therefore dependent upon a stable thorax for their efficient action (Fig. 2.7 a, b). The contractions of these two muscles would otherwise elevate the ribs instead of holding or moving the scapula. Likewise, the vast pectoralis major, which is involved in so many movements of the arm in action, arises from not only the anterior surfaces of the clavicle and sternum, but also from the cartilages of nearly all the true ribs, and even from the aponeurosis of the oblique abdominus externus (Fig. 2.8). The pectoralis would certainly elevate the rib cage were it not held in place from below.

To enable these muscles to function efficiently, the muscles of the abdominal wall must adapt their tension accordingly to hold the ribs down. The won-

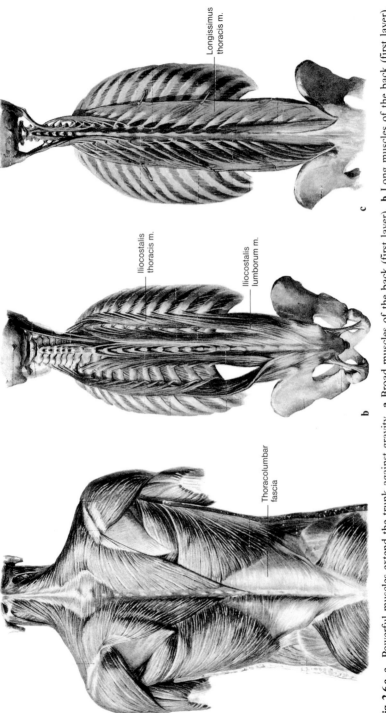

Fig. 2.6a–c. Powerful muscles extend the trunk against gravity. **a** Broad muscles of the back (first layer). **b** Long muscles of the back (first layer). **c** Long muscles of the back (second layer). Many of the long muscles have attachments to the angles of the ribs

Longissimus thoracis m.

Iliocostalis thoracis m.

Iliocostalis lumborum m.

Thoracolumbar fascia

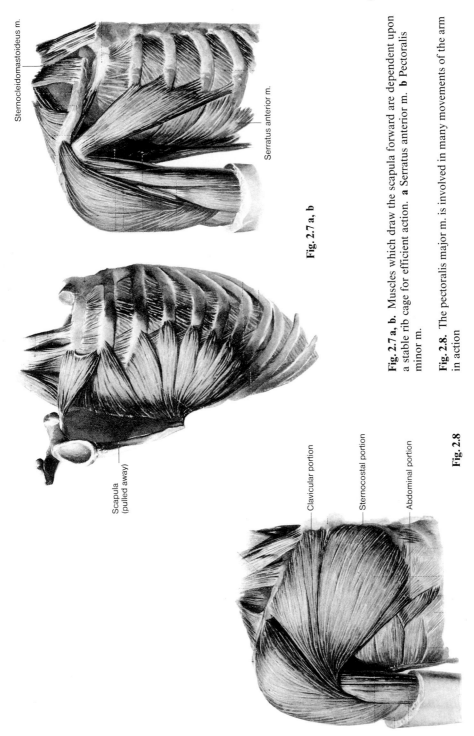

Sternocleidomastoideus m.

Serratus anterior m.

Fig. 2.7 a, b

Scapula
(pulled away)

Clavicular portion

Sternocostal portion

Abdominal portion

Fig. 2.8

Fig. 2.7 a, b. Muscles which draw the scapula forward are dependent upon a stable rib cage for efficient action. **a** Serratus anterior m. **b** Pectoralis minor m.

Fig. 2.8. The pectoralis major m. is involved in many movements of the arm in action

derful arrangement of the oblique abdominal muscles, particularly the external oblique which interdigitates with serratus anterior, allows for optimal counter-fixation of the ribs, as does the insertion of the rectus abdominis (Fig. 2.9). Without these muscle groups elevation of the rib cage secondary to extending the spine or lifting the arms would be inevitable (Fig. 2.10). All the muscles which act on the shoulder and enable it to be moved in so many complex ways are dependent upon the proximal anchorage provided by the shoulder girdle, which itself is dependent upon thoracic stabilisation. Such a fixation requires a constant and subtle interplay between the flexors and extensors of the trunk.

2.3.2.3 Abdominal Muscles

For the abdominal muscles to act efficiently they need a stable origin, which is either the pelvis, the thorax or the central aponeurosis, depending upon which part of the trunk is moving. Because origin and insertion are constantly changing during activity, the terms become difficult to define exactly. The pelvis is stabilised in lying, sitting and standing by the activity of the muscles around the hips, and in sitting and lying the stabilisation is helped by the weight of the legs themselves. Stabilisation of the thoracic origin for activities in which the abdominals contract to move or prevent movement of the pelvis requires selective extension of the thoracic spine. The muscles, particularly the obliques, cannot function efficiently when their origin and insertion are approximated, as they are when the spine is flexed with an exaggerated thoracic kyphosis.

There is a tendency to visualise the abdominal muscles as being situated solely on the anterior aspect of the trunk, perhaps because of the term 'stomach muscles' or the habit of beating proudly on that portion of the body when boasting of good athletic condition! From an anatomical point of view the muscles are actually situated laterally and posteriorly as well as anteriorly, the fibres of some extending right round to the back as far as the thoracolumbar fascia, which in turn is attached to the lumbar vertebrae. With regard to origin and insertion, the tendency is to describe the muscle fibres as running from pelvis to thorax. It is important to note that a large percentage of the fibres are, in fact, attached not to bone, but into an aponeurosis connected medially to the linea alba in such a way as to be continous with the aponeurosis of the opposite muscle (Fig. 2.11 a, b). The efficient action of the muscles of one side of the abdominal wall is therefore very much dependent upon the fixation or anchorage provided by the activity of the muscles on the other side, particularly for activities involving rotation of the trunk.

Rotation of the trunk is carried out by the oblique abdominal muscles. The activity is not unilateral, but requires the static holding of the contralateral muscles to stabilise the aponeurosis, so allowing the agonists to shorten and draw one side of the pelvis or thorax forwards. As Schulz (1982) explains: "Almost all the twisting movement is developed by the abdominal oblique muscles, with the various divisions of the obliques contributing about equally to the effort. The erector spinae are called upon in a maximum twist effort but they are not directly rotators of the trunk, despite what the anatomy text-books say.

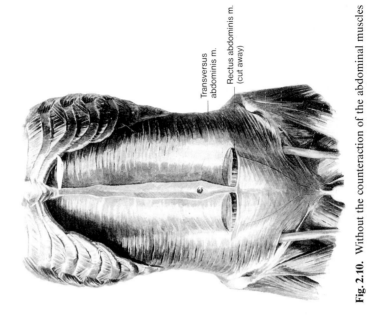

Transversus abdominis m.

Rectus abdominis m. (cut away)

Fig. 2.10. Without the counteraction of the abdominal muscles lateral elevation of the rib cage would be inevitable

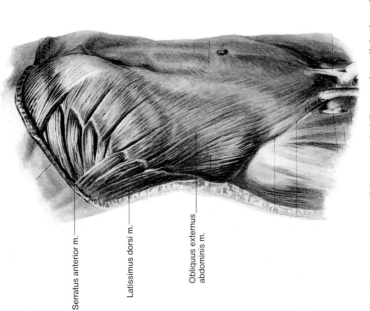

Serratus anterior m.

Latissimus dorsi m.

Obliquus externus abdominis m.

Fig. 2.9. Arrangement of the external oblique m. interdigitating with serratus anterior provides counterfixation of the ribs

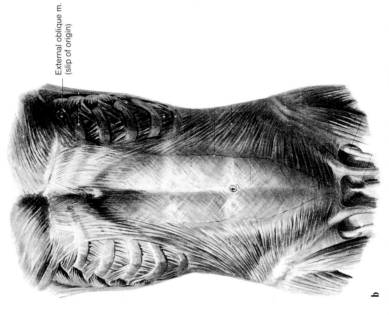

External oblique m.
(slip of origin)

b

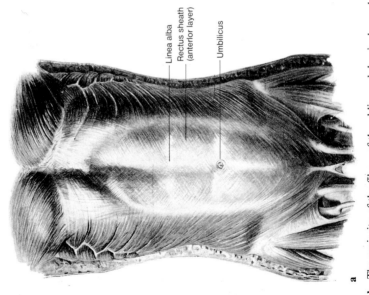

Linea alba
Rectus sheath
(anterior layer)
Umbilicus

a

Fig. 2.11 a, b. The majority of the fibres of the oblique abdominal muscles are attached to a central aponeurosis and not to bone **a** Obliquus externus abdominis m. **b** Obliquus internus abdominis m.

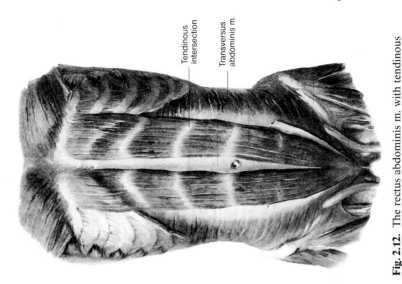

Fig. 2.12. The rectus abdominis m. with tendinous intersections. Shortening of the upper part without the lower is possible and vice versa

They contract in order to balance the flexion and lateral bending movements that necessarily develop when the abdominal oblique muscles contract".

It has sometimes been postulated that trunk rotation is the result of unilateral back extensor activity. In an electromyograph (EMG) study of axial trunk rotation (Donisch and Basmajian 1972), however, all subjects showed bilateral activity in the deep back muscles at the thoracic level, even though most rotatory movement takes place in the thoracic region. The bilateral back extensor activity would seem to support the hypothesis that the oblique abdominals are the prime rotators of the trunk, the extensors in the thoracic region acting to stabilise the thorax for efficient abdominal contraction.

The rectus abdominis does in fact run primarily from bone to bone or bone cartilage and is a prime flexor of the trunk. It is so constructed that its fibres are interrupted by fibrous bands or tendinous intersections and can contract in part, either the lower portion shortening while the upper fibres remain unchanged or vice versa (Fig. 2.12).

2.3.2.4 Respiration

Both the extensors and flexors of the trunk are directly related to respiration, inspiration being associated with extension and expiration with flexion. The spine does not move during the activity because of appropriate reciprocal tension in the antagonistic muscle groups. An excessive kyphotic position of the thoracic spine with its concomitant compression of the rib cage would reduce the volume of the lungs. The extensors of the thoracic spine act to ensure the size of the rib cage and also to provide a stable origin for the efficient functioning of the abdominal muscles during breathing.

Three groups of muscles are responsible for respiration: the diaphragm, the intercostal and accessory muscles, and the muscles of the abdomen. All three groups have inspiratory and expiratory function and work together in complex and co-ordinated ways. The abdominal muscles, including the rectus and transverse abdominis and the internal and external obliques, are usually described as expiratory muscles which augment the passive recoil of the lungs, particularly during forced expiration or deep breathing.

"The muscles of the anterior and lateral walls of the abdomen are the most important muscles of expiration" (Campbell 1955). But as Luce et al (1982) points out "the abdominal muscles also play a facilitatory role in inspiration in that their contraction tends to lengthen the diaphragm and diminish its radius of curvature, allowing it to generate a greater tension...". De Troyer (1983), describing how the abdominal muscles improve the ability of the diaphragm to generate pressure, writes that "since the abdominal muscles displace the diaphragm into the thorax when they contract, they indeed lengthen its muscle fibres and place them on a more advantageous portion of their length tension curve". As Sharp (1980) so clearly states: "The abdominal and accessory muscles also act as fixators or positioning muscles which adjust the configuration of the rib cage and abdomen in such a way as to optimize the efficiency of the diaphragm". Although the diaphragm is considered to be primarily a muscle of inspiration, it also plays a significant role throughout most of the breathing cycle. "Studies made of the diaphragm during passive expiration showed that electrical activity continued from inspiration into expiration. In some instances the activity continued through as much as 98% of expiration" (Murphy et al. 1959). In addition, Murphy writes that: "The presence of electrical activity during passive expiration suggests a braking action by this muscle to oppose the normal elastic forces of the lungs rather than the exertion of a true expiratory force".

It becoms obvious, therefore, that the abdominal muscles, play a significant role in normal respiration.

2.4 Types of Muscle Action

The muscles act on the trunk in three different ways, and as a result of the activity: (1) Movement occurs in a direction opposite to that of the pull of gravity (concentric muscle activity) (2) Movement which would otherwise take place due to the pull of gravity, or other forces acting on the body, is prevented (isometric muscle activity) (3) Movement in the direction of the pull of gravity is controlled by a braking action or 'paying out' of the muscles (eccentric muscle activity).

1. Movement in a Direction Opposite to the Pull of Gravity. From the moment when we get out of bed in the morning we change posture constantly and to do so must move our trunk in a direction opposite to the pull of gravity. We turn over in bed, we sit up from lying, come to standing from sitting, and grasp and lift objects from different surfaces all day long. When moving against gravity, the muscles on the uppermost side of the "tentacle" or the underside of the "bridge" shorten to move the trunk away from the earth. The speed of the movement alters the amount of muscle activity required. In general, the slower the rate of the movement, the more the muscle activity. In our daily life, the trunk is very often moved in a way which would fit the description of the "tentacle". We move it freely to bring our hands or our head into the required position, or our legs for that matter, for example when putting on our shoes, standing up and walking somewhere. Although the muscle activity is often described in relation to flexion or extension of the trunk, for functional activities these are usually accompanied by rotation and/or lateral flexion.

Basmajian (1979) considers that: "Man's so-called antigravity muscles are not so much to maintain normal sitting and standing postures as they are to produce the powerful movements required for the major changes from lying, to sitting, to standing". He explains, in addition, that "man is constantly challenging gravity by his continued wide range of postures, and great power is required only to achieve them".

2. Preventing Movement Which Would Otherwise Take Place as a Result of the Pull of Gravity of Other Forces Acting upon the Body. Muscle activity to prevent the trunk from moving towards the earth is required to maintain all postures and forms the basis of many balance reactions. When the arms are lifted, the trunk has to be held steady to counteract the weight of the long levers of the arms, and objects being held in the hands mean additional weight. Balance reactions involving the head, arms or legs require holding activity from the trunk. During respiration the muscles of the trunk act as fixators or stabilisers, resisting the force of the respiratory movements.

3. Controlling the Speed of Movement Taking Place in the Direction of the Pull of Gravity. Many activities of daily life require that we bend or lean forwards, backwards or sideways in a controlled manner to reach for objects or to place objects on a supporting surface. The muscles on the side of the trunk which is away from gravity control the speed of the movement as well as the range, by paying out or exerting a braking effect. The same applies when we bring a part of our body into a desired position, e. g. to lie down in bed, to bring our head forwards to eat or drink or to kiss a child. During expiration the braking effect of the diaphragm and the abdominals controls the flow of exhaled air and enables us to speak using sentences of a normal length.

The extensors and abdominals are constantly changing their mode of action according to the movement being performed or the posture being maintained. Interestingly, Caix et al. (1984), using the investigative techniques of histochemical analysis of striated muscle fibres and kinesiologic EMG of muscle function, found three functionally different populations of fibres and three categories of motor activity in the muscles of the abdominal wall. He and his coauthors propose the hypothesis that: "The three categories of recorded motor activity correspond to the contraction of three different populations of muscle fibres, i. e. slow fibres, fast fibres resistant to fatigue (fast resistant fibres) and fast fatiguable fibres". They postulate that the EMG signals of longest duration correspond to the slow fibres which have a tonic function, the signals of shortest duration correspond to the fast fatiguable fibres which have a phasic function and the signals of intermediate duration are produced by the fast resistant fibres which have a postural function.

2.5 Conclusion

"To move is all mankind can do and for such, the sole executant is muscle, whether in whispering a syllable or in felling a forest" (Sherrington 1947).

An action, reaction or interaction with the environment is only possible if a muscle contracts (Kesselring 1989). The muscles of the trunk are involved in all activities performed against gravity, and without a stable centre, movements of the extremities are possible only in mass synergies. The reciprocal innervation essential for selective movement of the limbs is dependent upon the degree of dynamic fixation provided proximally by both the flexors and exensors of the trunk.

3 Problems Associated with the Loss of Selective Trunk Activity in Hemiplegia

Hemiplegia, whatever its cause, is characterised by the loss of motor control on one side of the body. The typical inability to move the arm and leg, the development of spasticity in mass patterns and movement in stereotyped synergies have been clearly documented (B. Bobath 1978, Brunstrom 1970; Charness 1986, Davies 1985; Perry 1969). In addition, however, there is a most significant loss of selective activity in the muscles controlling the trunk, particularly in those muscles responsible for flexion, rotation and lateral flexion.

After onset of hemiplegia, the patient experiences difficulty in moving his trunk in relation to the pull of gravity, regardless of which type of muscle action is required. The abdominal muscles demonstrate a remarkable loss of activity and tone. In supine lying, the ribcage is drawn upwards and outwards and the shoulder girdle lies in an elevated position bilaterally, causing the neck to appear shortened (Fig. 3.1). The umbilicus is drawn towards the non-affected side. The entire abdominal wall has a hypotonic appearance, and the hypotonia is confirmed by the total lack of resistance to stretch on palpation (Fig. 3.2). In a sitting position, the lateral wall bulges loosely above the pelvis on the hemiplegic side with a loss of the normal contour of the waist to a greater or lesser degree (Fig. 3.3). In both sitting and standing positions, viewed from behind, the distance from the vertebral column to the lateral border of the trunk is greater on the affected side than on the sound side (Fig. 3.4). The resultant loss

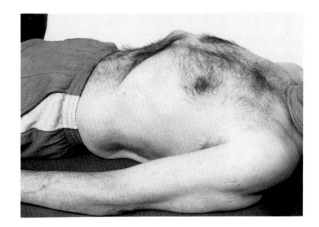

Fig. 3.1. In supine the rib cage is drawn upwards and outwards. The shoulder girdle lies in an elevated position, giving the neck a shortened appearance (left hemiplegia)

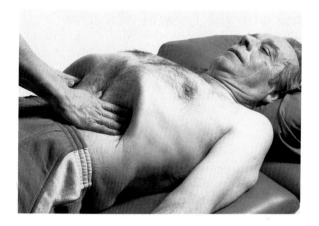

Fig. 3.2. Bilateral hypotonus of the abdominal muscles with lack of resistance to stretch (left hemiplegia)

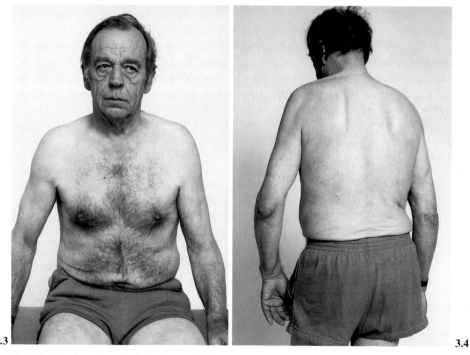

3.3

3.4

Fig. 3.3. The lateral wall of the lower abdomen bulges on the affected side with a loss of the waist contour (left hemiplegia)

Fig. 3.4. In upright positions the distance from the vertebral column to the lateral border of the trunk is increased on the affected side (left hemiplegia)

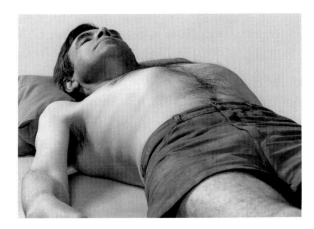

Fig. 3.5. Patient still demonstrates elevation of the rib cage with hyperactivity of the back extensors in supine 14 years after stroke (right hemiplegia)

of trunk control has far-reaching effects and is to a certain extent more disabling than the involvement of the arm and leg musculature, as the agility of children with extremity paralysis following polio demonstrates. The lack of proximal stabilisation influences the limbs profoundly in that the arm and leg can only be moved in spastic synergies. Distal spasticity is further increased as the patient tries to compensate for the loss of fixation when he attempts to move against gravity.

It is interesting to note that the patient's inability to control his trunk selectively closely resembles the stages of trunk control observed during the motor development of the normal baby and young child. It would seem that as a result of the hemiplegia the patient has been thrust back on to an earlier developmental level of motor function.

During normal development, extensor control of the trunk precedes flexor control, and the patient will likewise be able to extend his trunk actively at an early stage following the onset of hemiplegia. If he is not carefully treated, however, he will continue to use the more primitive extensor activity for all movements, and flexor control will not be attained. Such a situation is self-reinforcing in that the more the patient uses extension, the less will abdominal muscle activity be stimulated. The loss of flexor control can often still be observed even 10 or more years following stroke (Fig. 3.5).

3.1 Possible Reasons for the Bilateral Loss of Abdominal Muscle Activity and Tone

1. With the exception of the rectus abdominis, all the other muscles of the abdominal wall are attached by more than half to the central aponeurosis which is connected to the linea alba, and so each side is dependent upon the other for efficient action. The muscles on both sides are therefore im-

paired, and at an early stage of his disablement the patient begins to use compensatory muscles in order to move at all. He usually compensates by activating his back extensors and changing the position of his hips accordingly.

"The alienation of paretic muscles from an activity pattern occurs frequently. Only through specific training of control and co-ordination do those muscles again become incorporated as part of the normal activity pattern" (Kottke 1982 a, b). Without such specific training the muscles remain inactive, and recurrent inhibition may well set in and produce a "self-monitoring inhibition of motor neurons".

Usually, the abdominal muscles on the nonparetic side are affected as well, although not so drastically, due to the fact that no stable insertion is provided by the aponeuroses. As Perkins and Kent (1986), explaining the action of the transverse abdominals and obliques, write: "Because all of these muscles are paired, when contracted they pull in a tug-of-war fashion on opposite sides of the abdominal aponeurosis".

When activity is attempted, the contralateral side of the abdominal wall elongates, offering no anchorage for the contracting muscles. The patient may be able to contract the rectus abdominis as a whole in a mass pattern of flexion, such as when sitting up from lying, as both origin and insertion are more stable, being attached to bone, i. e. to the pubis below, to fixed rib cartilages and even to the xiphoid process of the sternum above.

2. In the early stages of hemiplegia the patient is obliged to use the more primitive extension of his trunk in order to be able to move his body at all. The back extensors are therefore in a constant state of activity, or even over-activity, which could well lead to reciprocal inhibition of the antagonists (Kottke 1975 a, b). Brooks (1986), referring to the lower limb in hemiplegia, explains how "the hyperactive extensors (deprived of supraspinal controls) tonically inhibit the physiological flexors which consequently are less spastic and more paralysed". The same mechanism could well apply to the flexors of the trunk.

3. The hemiplegic patient usually sits with his hips in some degree of extension and his thoracic spine flexed passively to compensate for his weight being behind his centre of gravity. In such a position the abdominal muscles cannot function effectively as their origin and insertion are already too closely approximated (s. Klein-Vogelbach 1989, personal communication).
When standing or walking the kyphotic position of the spine is also adopted by the patient to prevent his falling backwards.

3.2 Loss of Selective Activity

3.2.1 Muscles of the Trunk

Loss of selective activity in the various muscle groups of the trunk means that the patient is unable to stabilise his thoracic spine in extension while using his lower abdominal muscles (flexors) in isolation, as in walking, for example. Neither can he maintain the extension when using the abdominal muscles unilaterally for side flexion of the trunk or to rotate the side forwards.

3.2.2 Muscles of the Trunk and Limbs Acting Simultaneously

The patient is also unable to move his limbs in isolation without the activity occurring in a similar pattern in his trunk or move his trunk without movement taking place in his limbs. For example, when he sits up from lying, the legs will flex as well, making the movement difficult, if not impossible. In standing when the patient lifts one of his legs actively in front of him, his trunk will flex as well, and when he extends he leg behind him, his back extends.

3.3 Inability to Move in Normal Patterns

Due to the hemiplegia, and depending upon its severity, the adult patient's ability to move retrogresses to an earlier developmental level. Certainly in the first days following stroke, he feels "as helpless as a baby", as many a patient verbalises. He is unable to turn himself over in bed, come up to a sitting position unaided, and walking is frequently impossible for him. The regression refers only to motor function and in no way should the patient be considered or treated as a child. He is a thinking, feeling adult with a host of stored experiences and achievements and should be treated as such at all times. The comparison between the motor ability of the patient and that of the normal child will, however, help the rehabilitation team to analyse and treat the motor problems with more understanding and greater success.

3.4 The Most Commonly Observed Problems Seen in Relation to Normal Motor Development

As a result of the loss of trunk control, patients with hemiplegia will have difficulties, to a greater or lesser degree, with regard to the activities described below during their rehabilitation. The difficulties are more easily seen in certain positions or during specific movement sequences and will be described under headings referring to these. A difficulty observed in one movement or position will, however affect the performance of other normal activities as well. Breathing difficulties experienced will naturally restrict the patient's active participation in the entire rehabilitation programme.

3.4.1 Difficulties with Breathing and Speaking

With the rib cage held in a position of inspiration and the abdominal muscles flaccid and inactive, it is clear that the muscles of respiration cannot function efficiently (Fig. 3.6). Due to hyperactive extension of the spine, the patient's ribs with their long lever arm anteriorly are elevated together with the sternum. The elevation is accentuated further by the early development of hypertonus in the pectoralis muscle groups and by the patient activating these muscles as he attempts to move his hemiplegic arm by using the total mass pattern of extension.

The ribs are not held down from below by the abdominal muscles, and the configuration of the thorax is distorted. The movements of the rib cage will also be abnormal. Kolb and Kleyntyens (1937) recorded the movements of the chest with a kymograph and found, without being able to explain the findings, that "during hyperpnoea the movements on the affected side are increased out of proportion to those on the normal side. This increase persists longer than on the normal side and is noted in both spastic and flaccid hemiplegia". The difference between the two sides almost certainly can be explained by the insufficient activity in the abdominal muscles to "hold the ribs down", which Spaltenholz (1901) describes as being their main function.

The patient is not able to breathe out passively during quiet breathing as the elevated rib cage opposes the normal elastic recoil. When asked to breathe out he will usually press his lips together and blow the air out actively between them against resistance. Fugl-Meyer et al. (1983) found that "decreased expiratory force was a common denominator in stroke with hemiplegia or hemiparesis", and in a later study (Fugl-Meyer and Griemby 1984) that "abdominal electromyographic activity during forced expiratory manoeuvres appears constantly to be decreased".

Even patients who were known to have had extremely good respiratory function prior to stroke, with no previous history of lung disease, are short of breath during comparatively light activities. All the investigated patients in the study by Haas et al. (1967) had impaired respiratory function, and it is postulat-

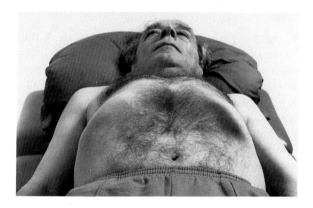

Fig. 3.6. The rib cage is held in a position of inspiration, preventing efficient respiratory muscle function (left hemiplegia)

ed that this impairment contributes to the fatigue which so often hampers the rehabilitation of hemiplegic patients.

Inspiration is also affected by the loss of stabilising activity on the part of the abdominal muscles. Due to abdominal wall laxness "respiratory mechanics are also interfered with by paradoxic inward motion of the upper thorax during upper intercostal contraction during inspiration" (Luce et al. 1982). The diaphragm cannot function efficiently, nor can the external intercostals as the ribs are already pulled upwards and approximated. "After the diaphragm the external intercostals are the next most important muscles of inspiration". They "function as if they were in a single sheet of muscle pulling all the lower ribs towards the first rib" (Perkins and Kent 1986).

In tests carried out on 20 patients with early flaccid hemiplegia, De Troyer et al. (1981) found that "in most patients a striking reduction in activity was observed during voluntary inspiration in both the intercostal muscles and the diaphragm on the side of the paresis". "In hemiplegia, moreover, forced inspiratory and expiratory volumes and maximum breathing capacity are also significantly reduced (Fugl-Meyer and Griemby 1984).

Not only does the patient tire easily during physical activity as a result of the reduced respiratory function, but he may have difficulty in speaking normally as well. The volume of his voice is reduced, and he is only able to use very short sentences, in a type of telegraphic speech. He may even rebreathe after each word as, for example, when counting or naming the days of the week. In order to use sentences of normal length it is necessary to be able to maintain a sound easily for about 12–15 s. The patient will often only achieve 5 s when tested.

3.4.1.1 Distorted Configuration of the Rib Cage

The fixed position of the ribs, or even rib cage contracture, has far-reaching effects on movements of the trunk itself, particularly flexion/rotation of the upper trunk. Flexion with rotation of the thoracic spine is a combination of movements which frequently occurs during functional activities, e. g. when lifting or placing objects to one side or in front and to one side. The ribs would block the movement, but they "possess the property of elasticity which allows them to distort during rotation of a vertebra" (Blair 1986).

With the ribs held in a fixed position from above, the instrinsic flexibility of their shafts as described by Schultz et al. (1974) is prevented from allowing the changes in the shape of the chest wall which are necessary for flexion, rotation and lateral flexion of the thoracic spine. Both active and passive movements feel blocked in all starting positions during therapy.

3.4.2 Difficulties Observed in Lying

In supine lying, because the rib cage is in a position of inspiration, the shoulder girdle is elevated, causing the neck to appear shortened. The umbilicus is drawn towards the sound side (Fig. 3.7 a). When the patient flexes his leg up towards him or his leg is placed in flexion by the therapist, the hip adopts a position of lateral rotation with abduction, the knee flexes and the foot supinates (Fig. 3.7 b).

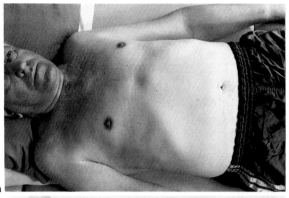

a

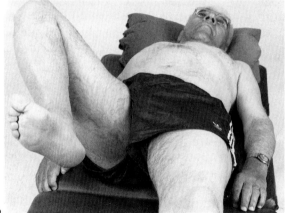

b

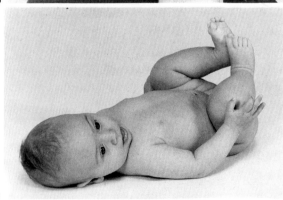

c

Fig. 3.7. a The umbilicus is drawn towards the sound side (right hemiplegia).
b The hip laterally rotates and abducts when the hemiplegic leg is flexed. The foot supinates (right hemiplegia).
c A normal 3-month-old baby shows a similar mass pattern of flexion of the legs. Typically the lower ribs are expanded, the shoulder girdle elevated and the neck very short

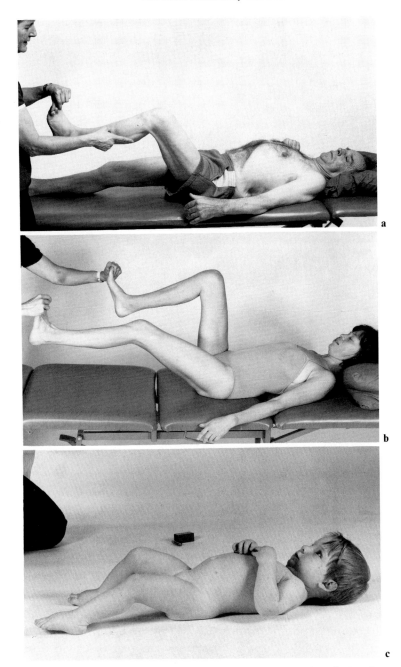

Fig. 3.8 a–c. Hip flexion accompanied by extension of the lumbar spine. **a** When flexing the hip actively, the patient attempts to stabilise his pelvis by pressing the sound leg down on the supporting surface (left hemiplegia). **b** When flexing both hips actively, lordosis increases and the abdomen protrudes (right hemiplegia). **c** A 9-month-old normal baby demonstrates a similar posture

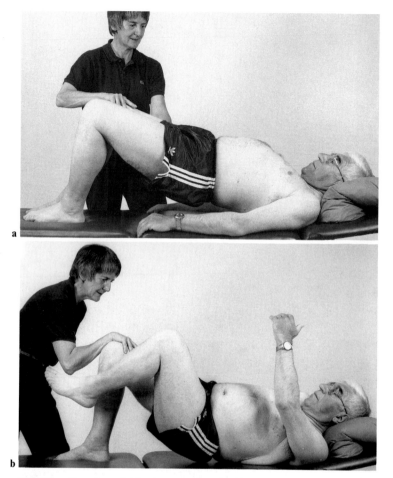

Fig. 3.9. a Forming a bridge by extending the hips and spine. **b** When the sound foot is lifted, the pelvis drops down on the ipsilateral side due to inadequate abdominal muscle activity (right hemiplegia)

As the Bobaths (K. Bobath and B. Bobath 1977) explain, the patient with hemiplegia is only able to activate his muscles on the affected side in one or two mass synergies, and these synergies, as seen for example in the young baby, are inadequate for functional activities. The patient is unable to adduct his flexed hip, or to move other parts of the leg selectively while the hip is flexed. Adduction of the hip in supine lying would require activity from the abdominal muscles to stabilise the pelvis. The young baby typically has a very short neck, his lower ribs are expanded and he flexes his legs in a similar pattern (Fig. 3.7 c).

When the patient holds his hemiplegic leg in flexion, the lumbar spine extends and he attempts to stabilise his pelvis by forcibly extending the leg on the

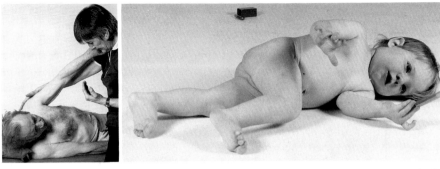

Fig. 3.10. a Turning towards the sound side. Without fixation by the abdominal muscles the ribs are pulled upwards instead of the head being raised (left hemiplegia). **b** A 9-month-old baby rests its head on the floor when rolling over to reach for an object

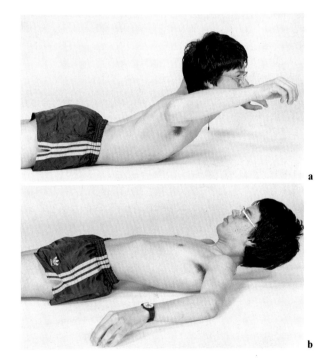

Fig. 3.11. a In prone lying, the patient is able to lift his head and shoulders using extensor activity (left hemiplegia). **b** From a supine position he is unable to flex his trunk to come up to sitting (left hemiplegia)

sound side, pressing the heel down against the supporting surface (Fig. 3.8 a). If both lower limbs are moved simultaneously the lumbar spine extends and the abdomen protrudes (Fig. 3.8 b). A baby 9–10 months old has the same posture (Fig. 3.8 c). Some patients blow out their abdomen forcibly in an attempt to compensate for the loss of stabilising abdominal muscle activity.

At an early stage the patient is able to extend his spine and hips and raise his buttocks off the supporting surface when lying with his knees and hips flexed to form a "bridge" (Fig. 3.9 a). At about 6 months a baby can often be observed making the same movement as it bounces its bottom up and down while lying on the floor. When, however, the patient lifts his sound foot into the air, the leg becomes a "tentacle" requiring activity from the abdominals to support it. The pelvis cannot be held level and sinks down on the sound side (Fig. 3.9 b). With insufficient tone and activity the oblique abdominal muscles are unable to suspend the bridge from above.

Rolling over on to his side the patient is unable to lift his head sufficiently against gravity, and the head righting reaction is inadequate. Lateral flexion of the neck to support the weight of the head and allow it to right is dependent upon a stable anchorage from the thorax. Without fixation from the abdominal muscles, the ribs are pulled upwards instead of the head being raised (Fig. 3.10 a). When the young baby starts to roll over on to its side to reach for an object, it will frequently rest its head on the floor for the same reason (Fig. 3.10 b).

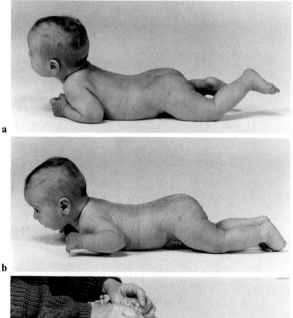

a

b

c

Fig. 3.12 a–c. In normal development active control of extension of the trunk precedes active flexion by far. **a** A 3-month-old baby raises his head in prone lying. **b** He can lift his head and shoulders without the support of his arms. **c** He is unable to flex his trunk to sit up, and his legs cannot extend selectively

3.4.3 Difficulties in Moving Between Lying and Sitting

In prone lying, the activity of the more primitive extensor muscles allows the patient to raise his head and shoulders from the floor without the support of his arms (Fig. 3.11 a). From a supine position, however, many patients are unable to come up to a sitting position unaided (Fig. 3.11 b).

Despite the size and weight of his head in proportion to his body, a baby can raise his head and shoulders from an early age (Fig. 3.12 a). He can even do so without pushing on his elbows (Fig. 3.12 b). Even with help, though, he is unable to come up to sitting, and holding his head flexed against gravity presents problems (Fig. 3.12 c). It will take a few years for him to achieve an adult pattern.

When the patient sits up with the therapist helping by holding his hands, he raises his arms to be able to use his more effective back extensors (Fig. 3.13 a). He has difficulty in keeping his affected leg extended on the floor to provide an anchor. A 10-month-old baby will also lift his arms as he too has more trunk

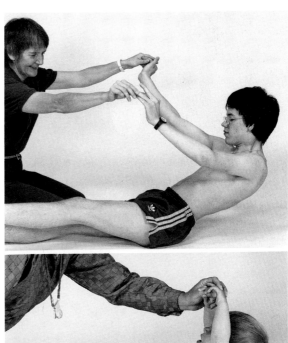

Fig. 3.13 a, b. Sitting up from lying with some help. **a** The therapist holds the patient's hands lightly to give support. The arms lift because the patient uses his extensors. His affected leg leaves the floor (left hemiplegia). **b** A 10-month-old baby also lifts his arms when his mother assists, and he cannot hold his legs down on the floor

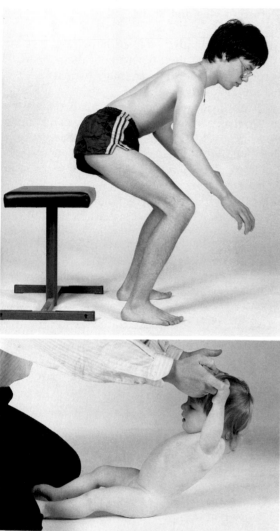

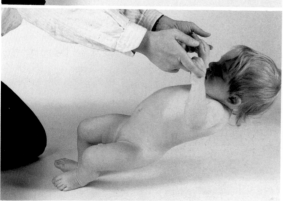

Fig. 3.14 a–c. Ability to use extension, but not flexion. **a** The patient can stand up from sitting using mainly his trunk and leg extensors (compare with Fig. 3.11 b; left hemiplegia). **b** A 9-month-old baby tries unsuccessfully to sit up using flexion. **c** The baby quickly brings her feet back and pushes up to standing using her extensors

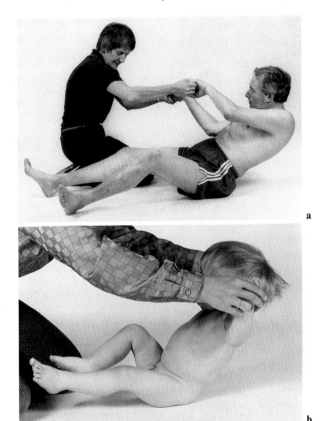

Fig. 3.15. a The patient has difficulty in coming up to sitting, even when the therapist pulls on his arms. He cannot extend his hemiplegic leg selectively when his trunk is flexing (left hemiplegia). **b** A 10-month-old baby has the same difficulty

extension control than flexion. His legs leave the floor, too, due to loss of selective activity between trunk and limbs (Fig. 3.13 b).

The patient finds it easier to stand up from sitting on a chair using the more effective extensor activity in both his trunk and his lower limbs, than to sit up from lying, which calls for flexion of the trunk (Fig. 3.14 a). A 9-month-old baby, finding the flexion tedious when pulled to sitting, often brings his feet back towards him and uses extension to come upright instead (Fig. 3.14 b, c).

Without selective activity between the trunk which is trying to flex and the legs which have to extend actively in order to remain on the floor, the patient cannot come up to sitting from lying even with help (Fig. 3.15 a). At 10 months the child can control the position of his head against gravity, but his legs flex and leave the floor too (Fig. 3.15 b).

When attempting to sit up with rotation with the hemiplegic side coming forwards, the arm flexes strongly in the spastic pattern of flexion with scapula retraction opposing the rotation. The patient's affected leg pulls into flexion as well, sometimes leaving the supporting surface altogether (Fig. 3.16 a). At 20 months, the child usually does not attempt to sit up with rotation, but if he

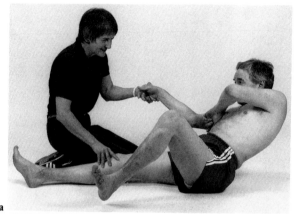

a

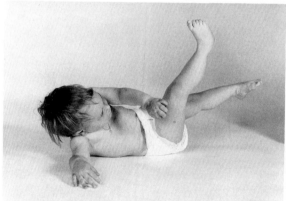

b

Fig. 3.16 a, b. Flexion of the trunk with rotation is even more advanced. **a** The patient is unable to flex his trunk and rotate towards the sound side when trying to sit up from lying. Both the hemiplegic arm and leg pull strongly into flexion (left hemiplegia). **b** A normal 20-month-old child attempts the movement, but fails. Her legs show total patterns of movement

does, his legs leave the floor as well and sometimes adopt a position very similar to the mass spastic synergies (Fig. 3.16 b). The arm also flexes, and the child is unable to bring his shoulder forwards with oblique abdominal control not yet sufficiently developed.

Even when sitting up with the sound side rotating forwards, the hemiplegic leg tends to flex despite the patient's conscious effort to maintain knee extension and keep the foot on the supporting surface (Fig. 3.17 a). The difficulty persists even when the patient is able to walk independently, but the gait pattern still shows abnormalities. At 3 years of age the child is not able to keep his legs extended and flat on the floor when sitting up with rotation either (Fig. 3.17 b). It must be remembered that even though he is already able to run around freely at this stage, the child's actual walking pattern is not the same as an adult's until he is seven years old (Okamoto 1973).

The patient who has difficulty in sitting up with rotation of his trunk, while at the same time extending his leg selectively will certainly still reveal problems of a similar nature when walking (Fig. 3.18 a, b).

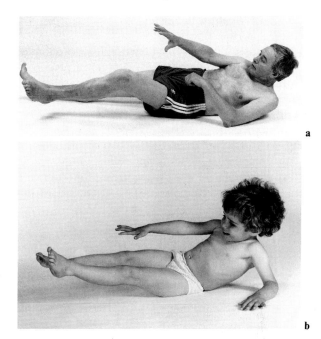

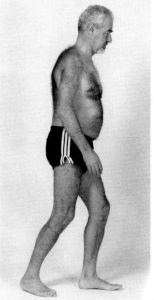

Fig. 3.17. a Even when rotating towards the hemiplegic side the patient is unable to sit up, and he cannot extend his hemiplegic leg while the trunk is flexing (left hemiplegia). **b** A normal 3-year-old child cannot sit up with rotation without using her arms for support

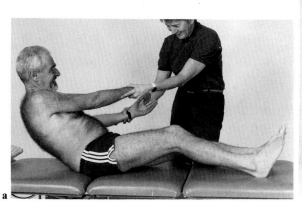

Fig. 3.18. a A patient who is able to walk long distances without aids still has difficulty in flexing and rotating his trunk towards the sound side (right hemiplegia). **b** His walking reveals similar problems

3.4.4 Difficulties in Sitting

The patient usually sits with his spine flexed and his neck extended, to a greater or lesser degree (Fig. 3.19 a). Such a posture is not due to weakness in his trunk extensors as is often mistakenly supposed (Fig. 3.19 b), rather the patient without adequate abdominal muscles and with his hip extended when he sits upright adopts the posture to prevent falling over backwards, which he would otherwise do (Fig. 3.19 c).

At 10 months a child also sits with his back rounded although he has excellent trunk extensors at this age (Fig. 3.19 d). He does so to keep his weight well forwards as he has neither sufficient abdominal muscle activity to prevent his falling backwards nor protective extension of his arms behind him should he

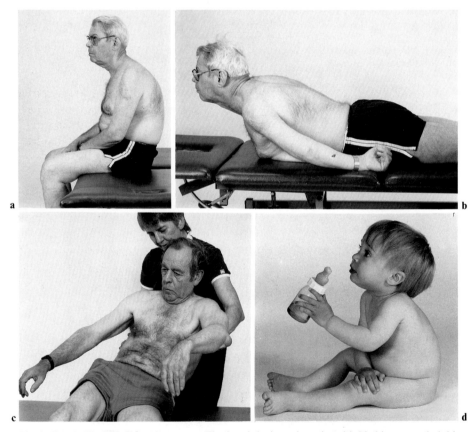

Fig. 3.19 a–d. Typical sitting posture. **a** The hemiplegic patient sits with his hips extended, his spine kyphotic and his neck extended (left hemiplegia). **b** It is erroneous to think that his trunk extensors are weak. **c** The kyphotic posture prevents his falling over backwards. **d** A 10-month-old baby adopts the same posture to avoid falling back as he also has too little abdominal muscle control

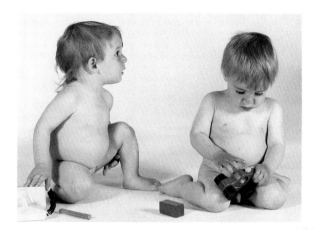

Fig. 3.20. Babies 9 and 10 months old adopt postures which allow them to extend their trunks without falling backwards

do so. Alternatively, he sits with his legs positioned in such a way as to provide a stable base, allowing him to extend his spine without being in danger of falling over (Fig. 3.20).

All balance reactions in sitting are adversely affected by the loss of selective trunk control. When the patient's weight is shifted sideways, his head cannot right if the abdominals cannot hold the ribs down. His trunk cannot shorten on the uppermost side away from gravity as lateral flexion involves all the abdominal muscles. His hemiplegic leg cannot abduct and extend to act as a counterweight as the pelvis is not able to provide a stable anchorage for the necessary muscles without the abdominals acting as fixators.

3.4.5 Difficulties in Standing Up from Sitting

The patient is unable to stand up normally from a sitting position because of inadequate selective activity in his legs and in his trunk (see Figs. 7.4, 7.5 and 7.9). If he stands up in an abnormal way, then his first steps when walking are automatically abnormal too (Davies 1985).

3.4.6 Difficulties in Standing

The patient with no abdominal control or insufficient activity in the abdominal muscles to support the long lever of his trunk against gravity would fall over backwards if he extended his spine and his hips simultaneously without support (Fig. 3.21 a). A 9-month-old baby, therefore, only stands when holding on to something (Fig. 3.21 b) or someone. It is interesting to note that the knees are hyperextended at this stage in his development. The abdominal muscles are required to tilt the pelvis up in the front and bring the hips into extension. The child's very lordotic lumbar spine ensures that his weight is kept well forward.

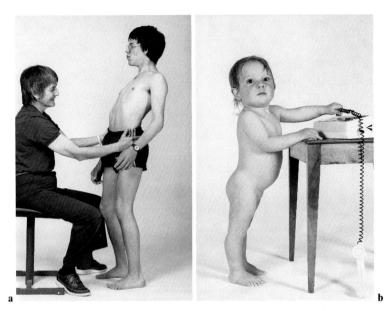

Fig. 3.21 a, b. Hip extension requires lower abdominal muscle activity. **a** Patient with poor abdominal control extends hips, but would fall over backwards if not held (left hemiplegia). **b** A 9-month-old baby only stands when there is something to hold on to, and she keeps her weight well forward. Her knees are hyperextended

The patient has to adopt an abnormal posture to keep his weight sufficiently forward. He often flexes his hips and knees to bring his entire trunk forwards, which the 10-11 months old child also does if he is not holding on or being held (Fig. 3.22 a, b). With the lack of abdominal control compensated for by 'holding on to something', both the patient and the baby hyperextend their knees, and the trunk is held in a more upright position (Fig. 3.22 c, d).

An alternative compensatory standing posture for the patient, and one which is frequently seen while walking, is the kyphotic thoracic spine (Fig. 3.23 a). By allowing his thoracic spine to flex, he ensures that his weight is not too far behind his centre of gravity. Normally "the position of the centre of pressure during standing fluctuates in a position slightly anterior to the vertical projection of the centre of gravity" (Murray et al. 1975). Hellebrandt (Hellebrandt 1938; Hellebrand et al. 1938, 1940; Hellebrandt and Braun 1939) reported that the mean position of the vertical projection of the centre of gravity was 5 cm anterior to the lateral malleolus. The patient's centre of gravity is usually too far back due to the hypertonus in the plantar flexors of his foot, the active plantar flexion of the foot as part of the mass extension synergy in the leg during weight bearing or his fear of falling forwards without adequate protective reactions. The child of 3 years stands with a similar posture, his thoracic spine kyphotic and his lumbar spine lordotic (Fig. 3.23 b). The overly lordotic position usually only disappears when the abdominal muscle activity is fully developed, many years later.

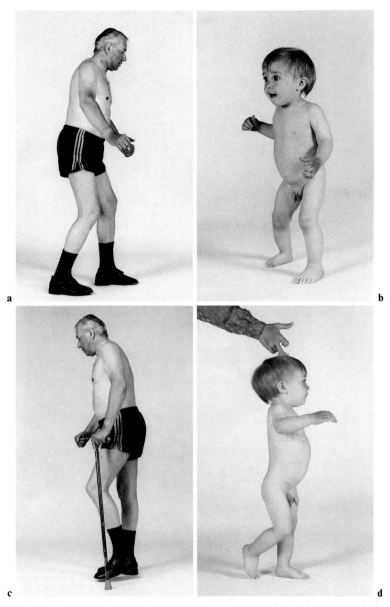

Fig. 3.22 a–d. Walking without sufficient trunk control. **a, b** To prevent falling backwards the patient (**a**) (right hemiplegia) and an 11-month-old baby (**b**) taking his first steps unaided flex knees and hips. The arms and hands of both flex to compensate for inadequate trunk stability. **c** With support, more extension (right hemiplegia). **d** With just a finger to hold extension becomes possible

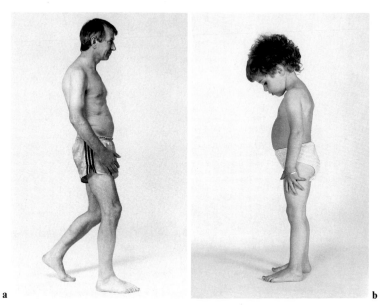

Fig. 3.23 a, b. Flexing the thoracic spine to keep weight forward. **a** Patient walks with typical kyphosis (right hemiplegia). **b** A 3-year-old girl with similar posture

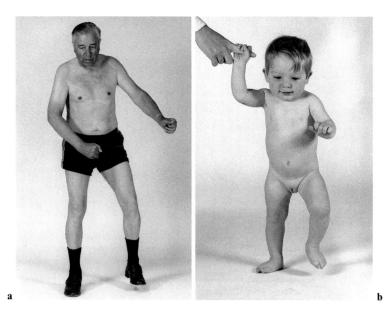

Fig. 3.24 a, b. Unable to transfer weight sideways. **a** Patient takes a quick short step to the side with the sound leg (right hemiplegia). **b** The 9-month-old baby must still hold on to something and also steps to the side. Arms and hands flex

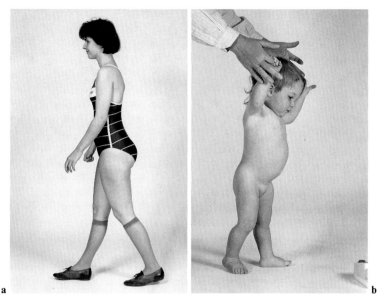

Fig. 3.25 a, b. Hyperextension of the knee in the stance phase due to inadequate lower abdominal muscle activity. **a** The pelvis remains tilted anteriorly and the hip does not extend (right hemiplegia). **b** Typical walking pattern at 9 months

3.4.7 Some Difficulties Observed in Walking

3.4.7.1 The Stance Phase

The patient is unable to shift his weight far enough over the hemiplegic leg. He therefore takes a rather quick short step with his sound foot which is placed well out to the side, like a protective step to regain his balance (Fig. 3.24 a). A child 9 months old, while enjoying walking when holding someone's hand, has a similar walking pattern (Fig. 3.24 b).

The patient whose lower abdominal muscles are inactive will hyperextend his knee as the pelvis is not tilted up in the front and his hip not extended (Fig. 3.25 a). A 9-month-old baby does the same when standing or walking with support (Fig. 3.25 b).

If the activity in the lower abdominals is not carefully and exactly trained together with selective extension of the lower limb, then the patient's knee will hyperextend during weight-bearing activities such as the stance phase of gait. In the study carried out by Knutsson and Richards (1979) "knee hyperextension was seen in all but one patient with hemiparesis during walking".

The problem is a very common one, even for patients who are walking independently and safely without any form of walking aid. With the knee hyperextended the ankle is never fully dorsiflexed, and hypertonus in the plantar

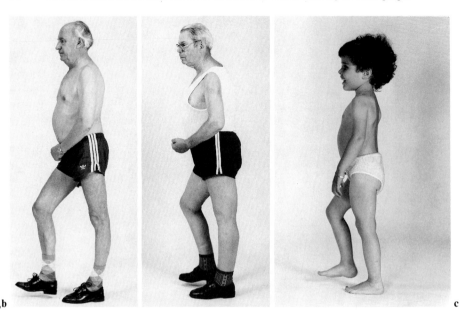

Fig. 3.26 a–c. No reactive step with the sound leg when the weight is too far back. **a** Hyperextension of the hemiplegic knee with plantar flexion of the foot (left hemiplegia). **b** Active lifting of the sound leg for the swing phase (left hemiplegia). **c** A 3-year-old child lifts her leg actively when stepping forwards

flexors will almost certainly be increased. Shortening of the achilles tendon may well be the result. As a result of the backward movement of the knee during the stance phase the swing phase of the sound leg will need to be active, instead of reactive as in normal walking. The patient has to flex his hip and knee in order to bring the foot forward, and the step length is reduced considerably and energy expenditure increased (Fig. 3.26 a, b). Because his hip moves backwards together with his knee, he does not bring his pelvis forward over the hemiplegic leg, and his weight therefore remains behind his centre of gravity instead of in front of it. The child of 3 years of age will be seen to have a similar walking pattern with no push off and an active swing phase (Fig. 3.26 c).

3.4.7.2 The Swing Phase

The pelvis on the hemiplegic side of the body drops down when the leg is not supporting it from below as it is not suspended from the muscles of the trunk above. The trunk side flexors do not take up the slack, as it were. The leg appears to be too long and at the initiation of the swing phase still has weight passing through it (Fig. 3.27). Often, extensor tonus is increased due to a positive supporting reaction, making initial hip and knee flexion difficult, if not impossible. The patient will have to use a compensatory mechanism to allow the hemiplegic leg to be brought forward:

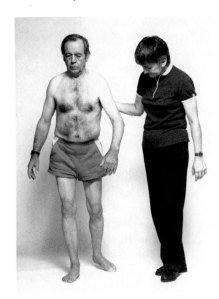

Fig. 3.27. The hemiplegic leg still bears weight at the initiation of the swing phase (left hemiplegia)

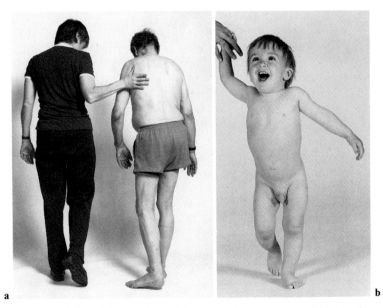

a   b

Fig. 3.28 a, b. Lateral shift of the pelvis over the weight-bearing leg to compensate for inadequate lateral flexors of the trunk. **a** Patient about to make a step with his affected leg (left hemiplegia). **b** A 10-month-old baby

- He shifts his pelvis laterally too far over the sound leg and, as a result, the affected leg often adducts as he brings it forward (Fig. 3.28 a).
- A baby, 10 months old, also shifts his pelvis laterally (Fig. 3.28 b).
- With difficulty in stabilising the thoracic spine, the patient is unable to transfer his weight over the sound leg and uses a mass pattern of flexion to take a step with the hemiplegic foot. The trunk flexes as he hitches the pelvis up with retraction on the affected side and circumducts his hip in order to bring the leg forward (Fig. 3.29 a). A 9-month-old baby uses a similar manoeuvre in order to clear the ground with his foot without transferring weight over the standing leg (Fig. 3.29 b).
- Some patients rise up on the toes of the sound foot to make more clearance for the hemiplegic leg. The leg is too long, not because of the lack of active dorsiflexion of the ankle, nor because the knee does not flex. The pelvis droops on that side, and the abdominal muscles acting as side flexors fail to support it from above (Fig. 3.30).
- Due to the effort of lifting the leg actively to bring it forwards, the arm pulls into the spastic pattern of flexion. Because the leg is flexing actively in a mass synergy, the patient's knee cannot extend at the end of the swing phase to bring the heel forward far enough for a normal step length. The patient's foot often supinates as a component of the total pattern of flexion, and he is at risk of spraining his ankle (Fig. 3.31 a). A child 3 years of age still has an active swing phase when walking (Fig. 3.31 b).

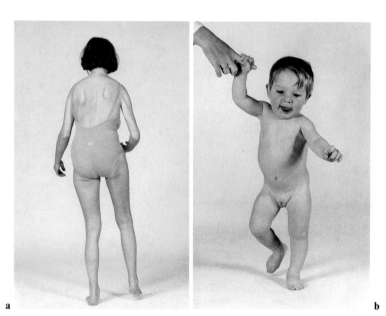

a   b

Fig. 3.29 a, b. Hitching up the pelvis with retraction and circumducting the hip. **a** Patient bringing her hemiplegic leg forwards (right hemiplegia). **b** A 9-month-old baby using a similar pattern

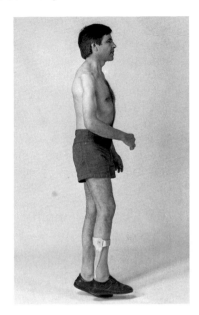

Fig. 3.30. Rising up on the toes of the sound side to allow the hemiplegic foot to clear the ground (right hemiplegia)

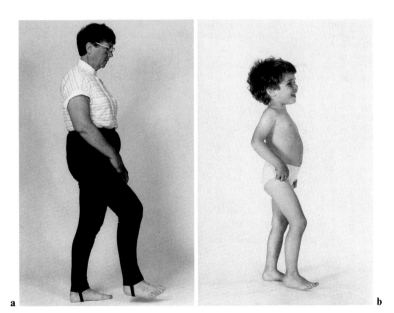

a   b

Fig. 3.31 a, b. Active flexion of the leg in the swing phase. **a** Using the total pattern of flexion to bring her leg forwards, the patient is unable to extend her knee at the end of the swing phase (right hemiplegia). **b** A 3-year-old child still flexes her leg actively when bringing it forwards

3.4.7.3 Slow and Effortful Walking with the Stride Width Increased

The patient walks with a broad base as far more stabilising trunk activity is required when the base is narrow. The speed of walking is reduced because the foot is placed to the side instead of forwards. "As compared to normal subjects of similar age, the hemiplegic subjects walked slower due to both shorter stride lengths and fewer steps per minute" (Dettmann et al. 1987).

The increased stride width, the slow speed of walking and the additional number of steps to cover a given distance make walking very effortful and uncertain (Fig. 3.32 a). When a baby first starts to walk without support, he will experience the same difficulties and usually sits down suddenly after taking a few steps (Fig. 3.32 b). He feels very unsure despite the broad base, as does the patient.

The baby taking his first steps will be praised for his courage and skill, unlike the patient, who will often be reprimanded for persistently using a cane or for being unwilling to walk at all. It should not be forgotten that the difficulties experienced by both the patient with hemiplegia and the baby in the normal course of his development are the result of inadequate selective trunk control and not due to any lack of motivation on the part of either.

Even as the patient's ability progresses and he can move around without aids, he still tends to walk with a greater stride width than normal and at a slower pace. The amount of effort he uses and his attempts to compensate for

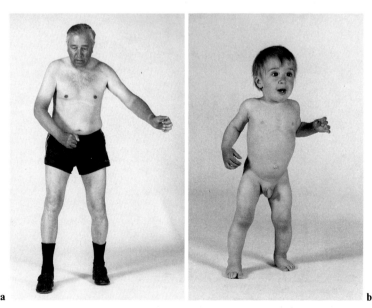

a   b

Fig. 3.32 a, b. Walking with a broad base. The patient steps more to the side than forwards with greatly reduced step length (right hemiplegia) (**a**); an 11 month old walking alone for the first time uses the same pattern (**b**). The arms of both compensate for loss of trunk stability

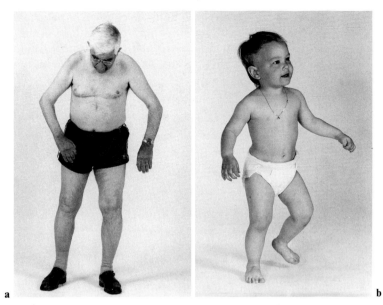

Fig. 3.33 a, b. Holding the head and shoulders in a fixed position to compensate for inadequate trunk control. **a** Patient hunches his shoulders and looks at the ground (right hemiplegia). **b** Child of 20 months of age tenses her arms and shoulders

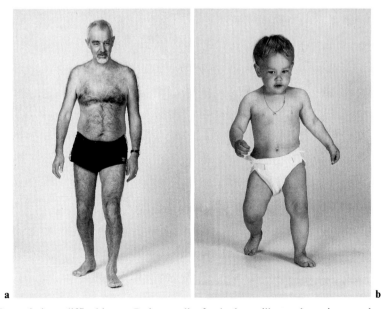

Fig. 3.34 a, b. Less obvious difficulties. **a** Patient walks freely, but still reveals an increased stride width, reduced step length, no push off and some tension in his arms (right hemiplegia). **b** A 21-month-old child has much the same pattern

inadequate trunk activity are evident in the position of his arms (Fig. 3.33 a). He also tends to keep his head in a fixed position and look at the ground in front of him. A child, 20 months old, also helps stabilise his trunk by holding his arms in a fixed position (Fig. 3.33 b). At an advanced level of walking ability,

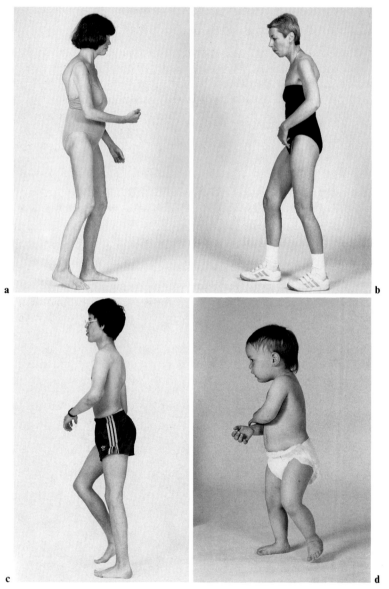

Fig. 3.35 a-d. Associated reactions in the arm due to effort or anxiety. Flexor spasticity is increased. **a** Initiating the swing phsae (right hemiplegia). **b** End of stance phase (left hemiplegia). **c** Lifting the sound leg (left hemiplegia). **d** Worried child, aged 20 months, looking for her mother

the difficulties may only be noticed because of some tension in the arms with loss of reactive arm swing, slight increase in stride width and, of course, reduced step length with resultant reduction of speed (Fig. 3.34 a). The same applies to the child in a stressful situation (Fig. 3.34 b).

3.4.7.4 Associated Reactions in the Arm

Whenever the patient is performing an activity which is effortful and for which he still has inadequate muscle control, associated reactions manifest themselves, particularly in the upper limb. Walking is a highly co-ordinated activity, requiring control from almost all muscles in the body. It is very common for the arm to become increasingly spastic when the patient walks unaided for any distance. The arm usually pulls up in the spastic pattern of flexion. The patient is quite naturally very disturbed by the effect the flexed arm has on his appearance. The increased tone in his arm hampers his ability to walk freely and easily still further (Fig. 3.35 a–c).

The hypertonus in the arm is like a barometer, informing the therapist of the patient's loss of proximal stability and selective activity. The young child, 20 months old, demonstrates a similar pattern in an anxious moment (Fig. 3.35 d).

3.4.8 Difficulties in Moving the Arm

The arm and hand can only be used functionally if the scapula and shoulder can be actively controlled in such a way as to bring them into and hold them steady in the required position. Proximal control is dependent upon selective trunk activity. The scapula can only be stabilised dynamically if the thoracic spine and the ribs can provide adequate anchorage or foundation for the relevant muscle groups.

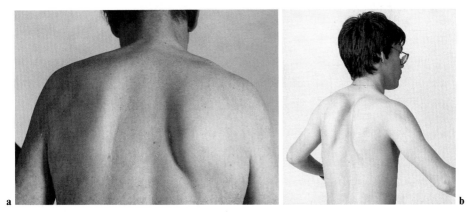

a   b

Fig. 3.36 a, b. Typical winging of both scapulae. **a** In sitting with the arms inactive (left hemiplegia). **b** When lifting the arms actively (left hemiplegia)

The patient has difficulty controlling the position of his scapulae (Fig. 3.36 a, b). The medial border of the scapula on both sides tends to swing away from the chest wall in all starting positions.

When moving his hemiplegic arm the patient attempts to stabilise the scapula by using a compensatory mechanism, often by fixing the contralateral shoulder blade or arm in a certain position (Fig. 3.37). Such fixation hampers normal bilateral use of the arms for performing tasks. The patient is usually able to move his arm better when lying supine as the scapula is stabilised by the weight of his body against the supporting surface. He is, however, only able to extend the arm with inward rotation of the shoulder as outward rotation requires abdominal activity to hold the ribs down (Fig. 3.38).

Bohannon and Andrews (1987) noted that some muscle groups around the shoulder were more affected than others. For example, the external rotator and abductor muscle strengths were more reduced than their antagonists. Both external rotation and abduction require rib-cage/scapula fixation.

When the patient raises his arm in abduction the hemiplegic side elongates, and the ribs on that side are pulled upwards. Although contracting actively the abductors of the shoulder can only move the arm in a mass synergy (Fig. 3.39 a, b). Even the activity of the sound arm is affected by the loss of stabilisation provided by the contralateral side of the trunk (Fig. 3.40 a, b).

When the patient moves both arms simultaneously, he is unable to prevent

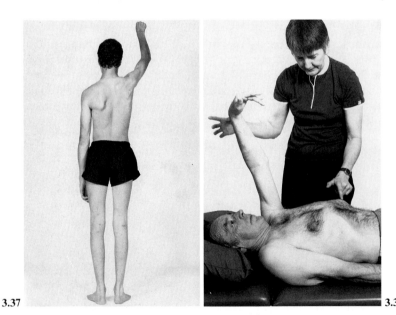

3.37   3.38

Fig. 3.37. Stabilising the scapula, using compensatory fixation of the shoulder blade on the sound side (right hemiplegia)

Fig. 3.38. Extension of the arm is only possible in a mass synergy, using adduction and inward rotation of the shoulder (left hemiplegia)

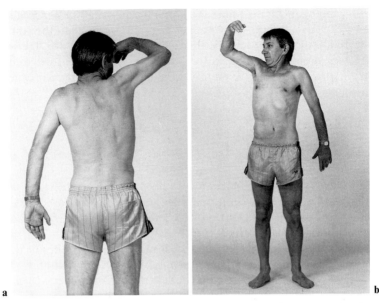

Fig. 3.39 a, b. Abduction of the arm in a mass flexion synergy (right hemiplegia). **a** The abductors of the shoulder work, but the ribs are not held down from below. **b** Without a stable foundation for the scapula the arm cannot be brought forward for functional use

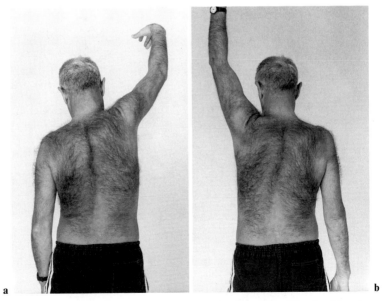

Fig. 3.40 a, b. Scapula control on both sides is affected (right hemiplegia). **a** The shoulder girdle elevates when the hemiplegic arm is lifted. **b** The trunk muscles on the hemiplegic side adjust inadequately when the sound arm is raised

the winging of his scapulae (Fig. 3.41 a). He usually extends his spine over-actively in his attempts to move the hemiplegic arm, and the resulting inhibition of his abdominal muscles further impairs the efficiency of the serratus anterior. Many patients actually lean forward from the hips in order to use extension of their trunk. Babies 9–10 months of age shows a similar lack of scapula stabilisation (Fig. 3.41 b).

3.5 Conclusion

All patients with hemiplegia have varied degrees of difficulty in some or all of the areas which have been described. When building a house everyone knows that a sound foundation is needed, and the patient, likewise, only improves his ability to move if the trunk offers such a foundation.

For successful rehabilitation with more quality of life for the patient, treatment must include all aspects, as one influences the other. If the activities described in the following chapters are carefully and exactly carried out, many of the patient's abilites will improve. Spasticity should always be inhibited before selective activity is attempted. With exact and continued treatment, improvement in motor control and recovery of active function does not necessarily cease 1 year after onset of hemiplegia as individual patients so often demonstrate (Fig. 3.42). The achievement of such improvement is most rewarding for both patient and therapist.

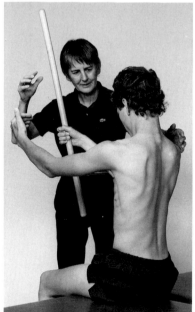

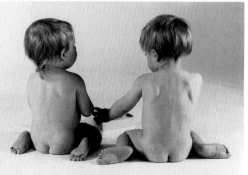

Fig. 3.41 a, b. Winging of the scapulae when moving both arms. **a** Impaired scapula control (right hemiplegia). **b** Lack of scapula stabilisation is normal in a 10-month-old baby

a

b

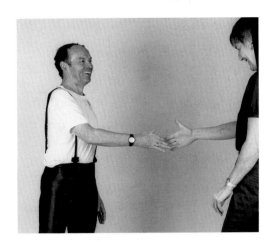

Fig. 3.42. Able to shake hands again at last, after 3 years of treatment following stroke (right hemiplegia)

Part II
Therapeutic Activities

For I know
he will not encumber me.
He ain't heavy.
He's my brother . . .

4 Activities in Lying

In the early stages after the onset of hemiplegia, when the patient has little control over the movements of his trunk, he can practise activities in lying in preparation for moving against gravity. Because the patient does not have to hold himself erect against the pull of gravity in this position, the activities can be performed with less extensor activity and effort, and the therapist is able to ensure that the movements are carried out accurately and economically. Not only in the early stages, but also in every stage of his rehabilitation, the patient will benefit from activities carried out in a lying position for the same reason. Functional activities such as walking (stance and swing phase), balance reactions, selective arm movements, breathing and speaking can be improved by the following activities.

4.1 Facilitating Breathing

4.1.1 Moving the Chest Passively

Due to the extension of his spine and the loss of tone in the abdominal muscles, the patient's ribs and sternum are frequently elevated, and so is his shoulder girdle (Fig. 4.1). Before activity is attempted the therapist should correct the

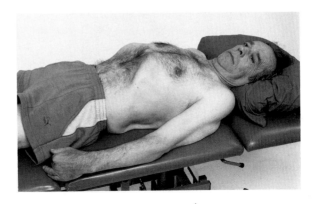

Fig. 4.1. Elevation of the rib cage and shoulder girdle in supine lying (left hemiplegia)

posture of the thorax. She stands at the head of the bed and places her hands anterolaterally over the patient's lower ribs. Leaning her weight forwards she moves the patient's ribs downwards and medially, to regain their normal position passively (Fig. 4.2). It is useful for the therapist to hold the thorax in the normal position for the patient while he continues to breath quietly. With the ribs in the corrected posture diaphragmatic breathing will often take place spontaneously, so activating the required muscles.

4.1.2 Assisting Expiration

Standing beside the patient the therapist assists the movement of expiration by placing her hands on either side of his thorax and pressing downwards and inwards. The patient is asked to make a long steady sound as he exhales (Fig. 4.3). At the end of expiration he can also try to hold his ribs actively in the corrected position of expiration when the therapist reduces the amount of assistance she is giving.

4.1.3 Facilitating Diaphragmatic Breathing

The therapist places her hands over the patient's lower ribs and brings them passively down and medially into the corrected position (Fig. 4.4a,b). With the fingers and thumb of one hand she maintains the corrected position of the ribs and asks the patient to breath quietly, using her other hand to indicate the rise and fall of the abdomen during inspiration and expiration (Fig. 4.5).

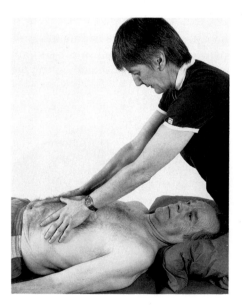

Fig. 4.2. Correcting the position of the patient's thorax passively (left hemiplegia)

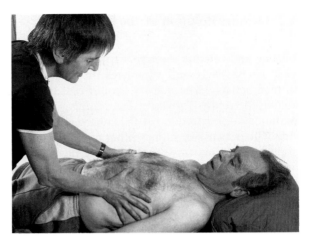

Fig. 4.3. Assisting expiration. With his head well supported on a pillow, the patient produces a long, steady vowel sound (left hemiplegia)

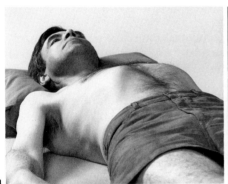

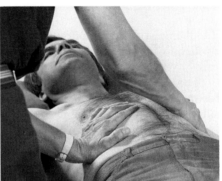

a   b

Fig. 4.4. **a** Over-active extension of the spine holds the rib cage in a position of forced inspiration (right hemiplegia) **b** Correcting the position prior to the facilitation of normal breathing patterns (right hemiplegia)

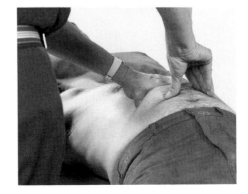

Fig. 4.5. Facilitating diaphragmatic breathing. The therapist holds the patient's ribs down with one hand, while assisting the breathing movement with the other (right hemiplegia)

4.2 Flexion/Rotation of the Upper Trunk

Flexing and rotating the upper trunk inhibits spasticity in the limbs when carried out passively and stimulates the oblique abdominal muscles when performed actively. The activity should first be carried out so that the patient's sound side rotates forwards. The resulting rotation of the trunk inhibits the hypertonus in preparation for the subsequent forward movement of the affected side. The patient lies supine either in bed or on a plinth with his legs extended, abducted and outwardly rotated. The position of the legs stabilises the pelvis and ensures that the movement occurs in the trunk. The therapist's support and facilitation is similar, whether the sound or hemiplegic side is being brought forwards, only differing in that she will need to give more assistance when the patient is flexing and rotating towards his sound side as the over-activity in the retractors of the trunk will oppose the movement.

4.2.1 Assisting Passive Movement

The therapist stands beside the patient facing his trunk. She rests the patient's furthermost arm on her shoulder and places her hands over his scapula, one directly over the other, with the hand nearest his head being uppermost.

The patient relaxes completely as the therapist draws the side of his thorax forwards and in the direction of his contralateral hip, by shifting her weight sideways. She instructs the patient to allow the movement to take place without any resistance and to leave his head lying on the pillow (Fig. 4.6). If the patient is very stiff or over-active, the trunk may rotate only in extension and the desired activity not be achieved (Fig. 4.7a). The therapist should observe the

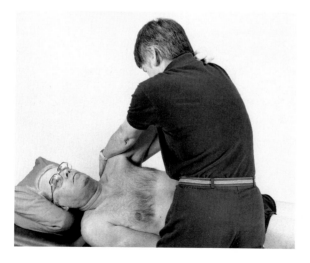

Fig. 4.6. Passive flexion/rotation of the thorax. The patient's head remains on the pillow (left hemiplegia)

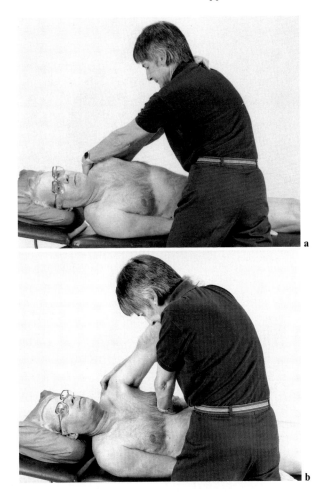

Fig. 4.7. Ensuring flexion of the thoracic spine. **a** Careful observation of the chest reveals that the spine is extending instead of flexing (left hemiplegia). **b** The therapist presses downwards and medially on the chest wall to achieve flexion (left hemiplegia)

movement and position of the chest carefully and, if necessary, use one of her hands to give a downward pressure over his sternum or lower ribs to ensure the flexion component of the upper trunk rotation (Fig. 4.7b). The passive procedure is continued until no resistance is felt, either to the flexion or to the rotation.

4.2.2 Facilitating Active Movement

The therapist moves the upper trunk into the fullest degree of flexion with rotation which is possible, and then asks the patient to lift his head. She assists the movement of his head with one hand, placing it in the correct position so that

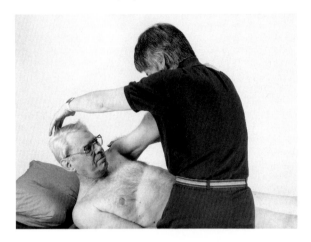

Fig. 4.8. The patient holds the position of his trunk actively and his head is guided into the correct position. The therapist reduces the amount of support (left hemiplegia)

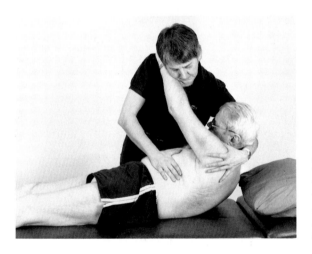

Fig. 4.9. Giving additional support to the flexion, rotation and side flexion of the trunk. The therapist presses the ribs downwards and medially and holds the patient's arm in place with her head (left hemiplegia)

his chin is pointing towards the middle of his chest, and his head held actively with some lateral flexion towards the uppermost side (Fig. 4.8).

The therapist encourages the patient to hold the position of his trunk and head actively as she gives less and less support with the hand which is behind his scapula.

Should the movement still be difficult for the patient, or to correct the position and increase the amount of trunk side flexion, the therapist can give additional support. She places her arm round behind his shoulders and uses her hand to guide his moving shoulder down towards his feet. Her arm also helps to bring his head into the correct position. Her other hand presses down over the patient's lower ribs, assiting the action of the abdominal muscles on that side (Fig. 4.9). The side flexion of the trunk is important as the lateral movement against gravity recruits almost all the abdominal muscles actively.

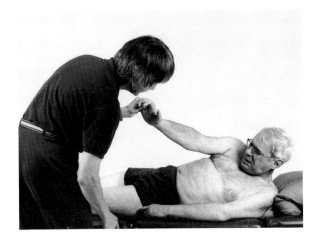

Fig. 4.10. Active flexion/rotation of the upper trunk with minimal assistance (left hemiplegia)

When moving the affected side forwards the therapist may need to support the hemiplegic arm to prevent it from falling from her shoulder. Usually her arm will provide sufficient fixation, but if not, she can hold his arm in place with her cheek at first, by flexing her neck sideways. As the trunk rotation is repeated, however, the muscle tone in the whole upper extremity is inhibited and his arm will remain resting on her shoulder. The movement is practised towards both sides until the patient requires only minimal guidance from the therapist (Fig. 4.10).

4.3 Retraining Active Protraction of the Scapula with Activation of the Oblique Abdominal Muscles

Many patients have difficulty stabilising the scapula against the wall of the thorax when the hemiplegic arm is raised (Fig. 4.11 a). The correct activity must be carefully trained in order to avoid compensatory movements being used (Fig. 4.11 b).

With the patient lying supine the therapist depresses his lower ribs medially on his sound side. She then places his extended arm in 90° of flexion with outward rotation at the shoulder and asks him to hold it there, without letting his ribs move laterally again (Fig. 4.12). The patient can move his arm carefully into abduction and back again, but only as far as he is able to while actively holding his ribs in place. The therapist then performs the same movement with the hemiplegic arm. The patient is asked to breathe gently without losing control of his arm or allowing his ribs to elevate. The small movement of the ribs against the contracted oblique abdominal muscles stimulates their increased activity (Fig. 4.13).

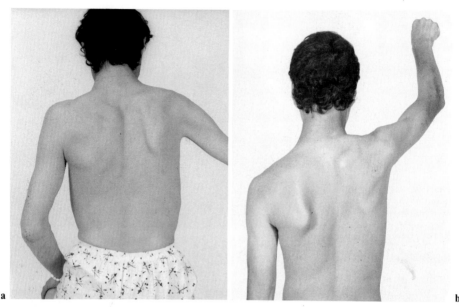

Fig. 4.11. a Typical loss of scapula control when the hemiplegic arm is raised (right hemiplegia). **b** Compensatory stabilisation of the scapula using the contralateral shoulder girdle (right hemiplegia)

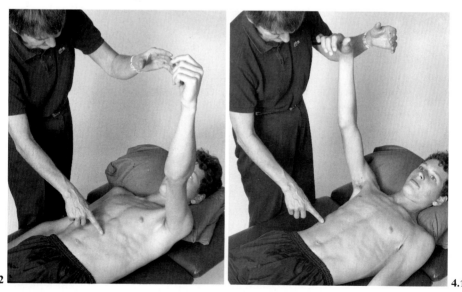

Fig. 4.12. Holding the ribs down actively when the sound arm is placed in a vertical position (right hemiplegia)

Fig. 4.13. Holding the ribs actively when the hemiplegic arm is held at 90° flexion of the shoulder. The patient breathes gently while the ribs remain in position (right hemiplegia)

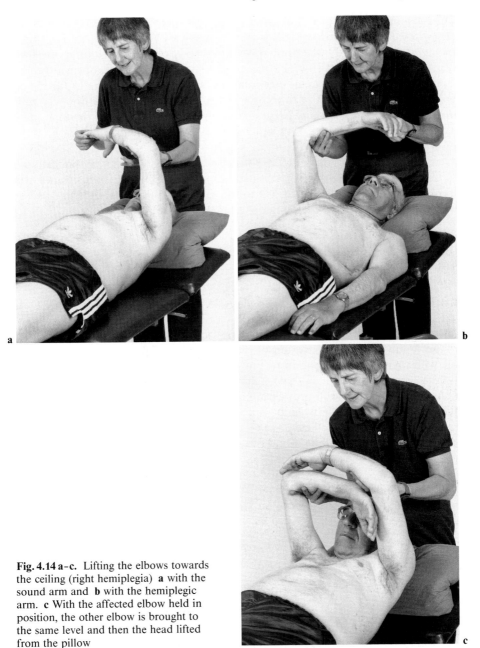

Fig. 4.14 a–c. Lifting the elbows towards the ceiling (right hemiplegia) **a** with the sound arm and **b** with the hemiplegic arm. **c** With the affected elbow held in position, the other elbow is brought to the same level and then the head lifted from the pillow

4.3.1 Lifting the Elbows into the Air

The patient lies supine, and the therapist holds his sound arm lightly and moves it into the air. The shoulder and elbow remain flexed at an angle of 90°.

The movement is repeated, the patient being instructed to bring the point of his elbow towards the ceiling (Fig. 4.14a). The same movement is carried out with the hemiplegic arm, the therapist supporting its weight and position more firmly if necessary (Fig. 4.14b). The movement should be carried out gently and carefully to avoid the patient extending his spine as he attempts to lift his elbow. The flexed position of the elbow eliminates over-activity of the pectoralis muscle group, which usually occurs if the arm is held straight in the total mass extension synergy. The patient's head remains lying in a relaxed position on the pillow.

When the patient is able to raise his elbows alternately and rhythmically into the air without excessive effort, the therapist asks him to keep his sound arm in place as he lifts the affected one to the same level. He then lifts his head as well without his elbows changing position (Fig. 4.14c).

4.4 Rolling to Prone

4.4.1 Rolling Towards the Hemiplegic Side

Due to loss of active flexor control of the trunk, patients will usually roll over to the prone position in an extensor pattern, starting the movement by pushing off with their sound leg and arm (Fig. 4.15). Active rolling from a supine position to lying on the side and back again using active flexion of the trunk can be facilitated and used to improve trunk control for patients in all stages of their rehabilitation. The activity can be practised on a bed, a mat on the floor, a high mat or two plinths placed side by side. It should not be attempted on a narrow plinth as the patient will be afraid of falling off it and will not move freely as a result.

The therapist kneels beside the patient cradling his hemiplegic arm under her arm against her body. Her hand supports his humerus from below so that his shoulder is protected (Fig. 4.16). She adjusts the range of movement so that no pain is elicited.

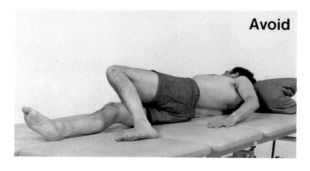

Avoid

Fig. 4.15. Patient demonstrating typical pattern for rolling over, using extension of the sound side (right hemiplegia)

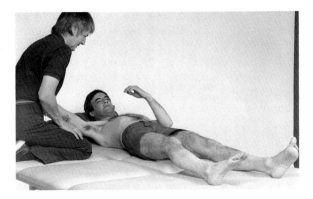

Fig. 4.16. Starting position for facilitating rolling towards the affected side (right hemiplegia)

The patient is then asked to lift his sound arm and leg upwards and forwards towards the therapist, without pushing off with his foot from the plinth behind him (Fig. 4.17 a). With a controlled movement he brings his leg gently on to the plinth in front of him, so that it comes to rest with the whole lower leg supported and not just the big toe pressing against the surface. The patient's head remains supported on a pillow at first, until he can roll onto his side and back again correctly.

The patient returns to the supine position by lifting his leg in abduction away from the plinth, rolling his trunk back, and only then lowering his extended leg slowly to the supporting surface (Fig. 4.17 b). In this way increased holding activity of the abdominal muscles is stimulated.

Once the patient has learned the movement sequence, he ist asked to lift his head from the pillow and hold it actively while rolling from a supine position to the affected side. The head is raised to initiate the movement and rotates in the direction towards which he is rolling (Fig. 4.17 c). When returning to the supine position the head is held actively until the leg has been lowered to the supporting surface (Fig. 4.17 d).

When the patient can roll onto his side and back again without undue effort, the therapist gives less support. She facilitates the movement by merely guiding his head into the correct position and drawing his sound hand forward (Fig. 4.18 a). The patient leaves his hemiplegic arm lying on the plinth and voluntarily inhibits the pull into flexion as he returns to a supine position (Fig. 4.18 b). Finally, he reproduces the whole movement sequence unaided (Fig. 4.18 c).

The therapist can then facilitate rolling right over to the prone position. She draws his sound hand forwards and, with her other hand, helps his hemiplegic arm to remain elevated. The neck extends when the patient has turned over. The sound leg remains in the air until the roll has been completed, the activity changing to extension of both trunk and hip as he reaches the prone stage (Fig. 4.19).

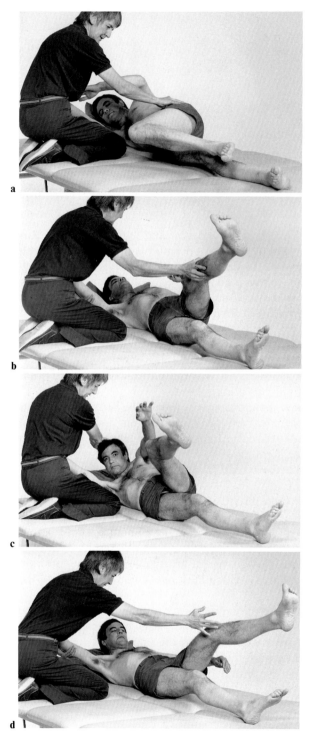

Fig. 4.17 a–d. Facilitating rolling towards the hemiplegic side (right hemiplegia). **a** With his head resting on the pillow, the patient lifts his sound leg upwards and forwards without pushing off with his foot. **b** He lowers his leg slowly as he returns to supine lying. **c** The patient lifts his head and then brings his sound leg and arm forwards as he turns over. **d** He holds his head actively as he returns to supine lying and lowers his leg slowly

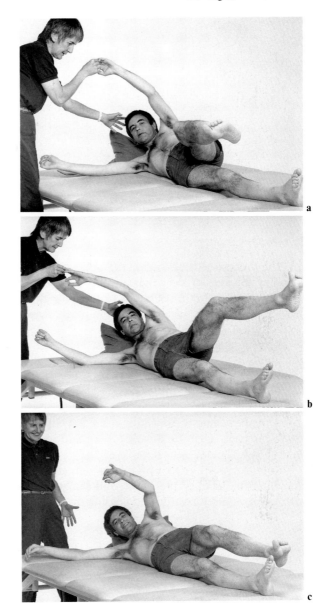

Fig. 4.18 a–c. Rolling towards the hemiplegic side with less assistance (right hemiplegia). **a** The patient lifts his head from the pillow and brings his leg forwards actively and the therapist guides his sound hand. **b** Returning slowly to the supine position with only minimal support. **c** Rolling over unaided. The patient does not allow his hemiplegic arm to pull into flexion

4.4.2 Rolling Towards the Sound Side

The untrained patient will usually turn onto his sound side by extending his head against the pillow or surface and use his back extensors to bring the extended hemiplegic leg forwards (Fig. 4.20).

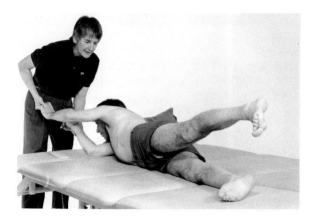

Fig. 4.19. Rolling right over to prone

The therapist kneels beside the patient at his sound side and assists him in bringing the side of his pelvis and his leg forward in a more normal way. Because she needs both her hands to facilitate the movement, the patient clasps his hands together, bringing the hemiplegic arm forward with the help of the sound one (Fig. 4.21 a).

Returning to supine, the therapist helps the patient lift his affected leg off the plinth and asks him to lower it slowly, but not until he is on his back again (Fig. 4.21 b).

When the patient is able to bring his leg forwards unaided, the therapist can facilitate the movement by drawing the hemiplegic hand forwards. She can also guide the head into the position of flexion with rotation (Fig. 4.22 a). As he rolls on to his back again he lowers his leg and head slowly to the supporting surface (Fig. 4.22 b).

Rolling right over to a prone position can then be facilitated. The therapist stands at the head of the plinth and facilitates the movement by drawing the hemiplegic hand forwards and guiding the head through flexion/rotation to ex-

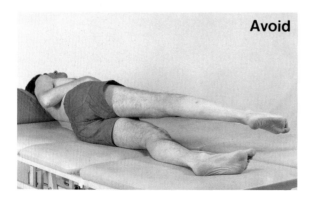

Avoid

Fig. 4.20. Patient demonstrating unwanted pattern when rolling over towards the sound side, using extension (right hemiplegia)

tension as the patient comes into the prone position. The patient is asked to hold his leg in the air until he has turned over completely (Fig. 4.23 a, b).

Rolling from supine to prone lying requires control of the trunk in flexion with rotation, extension and lateral flexion. Head righting reactions are also stimulated, and due to the rotation of the trunk, the distal spasticity in the arm is reduced. Correct rolling will improve the patient's ability to walk and can be used at any stage of the rehabilitation. The amount of support and facilitation decreases as the patient's control increases.

4.5 Flexion/Rotation of the Lower Trunk

The movement should be performed first towards the hemiplegic side. The tone in the hemiplegic side is thus inhibited by the rotation of the trunk and allows the movement to take place more freely to the other side afterwards.

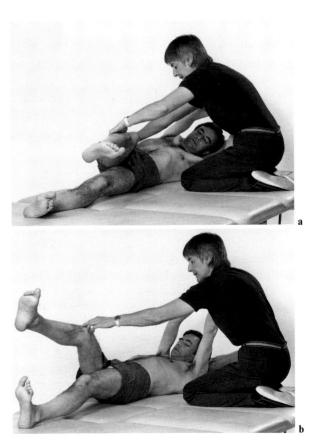

Fig. 4.21 a, b. Facilitating rolling to the sound side (right hemiplegia). **a** The patient's hands are clasped together and the therapist supports the hemiplegic leg. **b** The hemiplegic leg is lowered slowly to the surface when the patient returns to supine

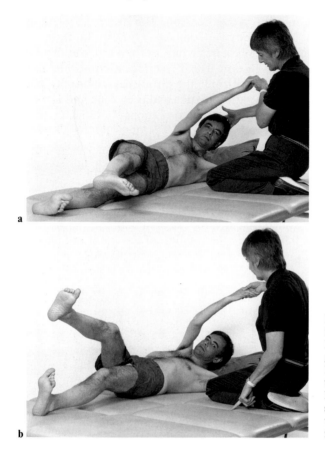

a

b

Fig. 4.22 a, b. Rolling to and from the sound side with less support (right hemiplegia). **a** The patient brings his hemiplegic leg forwards actively. The therapist guides his head into the correct position. **b** Returning to supine without the arm pulling into flexion

With the patient lying in a relaxed supine position, the therapist flexes both his legs so that the angle at the hips is approximately 90°. She asks the patient to relax completely without trying to assist her and rests his knees against her body in such a way that he does not need to hold their weight at all (Fig. 4.24a). By bending her knees, the therapist rotates the patient's lumbar spine, taking care that the rotation does not occur in the upper thoracic spine.

Placing one of her hands over the patient's sacrum and supporting his legs against her body with her upper arm, she transfers her weight sideways and moves his pelvis passively by flexing his lumbar spine. With her other hand she holds his rib cage down, and her index finger and thumb indicate the fulcrum around which the movement should take place. Seen from above, the point would be approximately at the level of the navel (umbilicus). The amount of flexion at the patient's hips does not change as the therapist draws the pelvis forwards. It is as if she was drawing his coccyx through between his legs. Should the patient's arm obstruct the movement, his elbow can be flexed and his hand laid upon his chest (Fig. 4.24b). When the passive movement is possi-

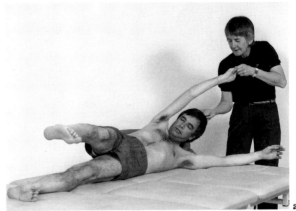

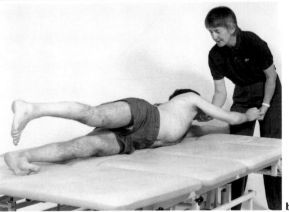

Fig. 4.23 a, b. Rolling right over to prone towards the sound side (right hemiplegia). **a** Neck and trunk flexion with rotation at first. **b** Neck and trunk extension with assistance

ble without any resistance being felt, the therapist asks the patient to help her actively, but gently, by contracting his lower abdominal muscles. The movement reduces the overactivity of the extensors of the lower back, allowing the abdominals to contract, and also inhibits extensor spasticity in the entire lower extremity.

4.6 Activating the Oblique Abdominal Muscles in Crook Lying

In crook lying, i. e. with his feet supported on the plinth so that his hips and knees are flexed, the patient crosses one leg over the other and rests the uppermost leg on the one below. The therapist facilitates abduction and adduction of the underneath leg in a smooth and rhythmic way and asks the patient to move actively with her. The patient's thorax remains motionless on the plinth and the moving legs activate the oblique abdominal muscles (Fig. 4.25a,b). The move-

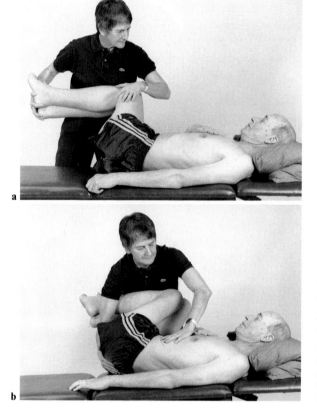

Fig. 4.24 a, b. Passive flexion/rotation of the lower trunk (left hemiplegia). **a** The patient's legs are totally supported against the therapist's body, and he relaxes completely. **b** With one hand over the patient's sacrum, the therapist gently flexes the lower lumbar spine. Her other hand stabilises the thorax

ment is repeated with the other leg crossed over, and the therapist gives less and less assistance (Fig. 4.26). The movement demands far more active control when the patient raises his sound arm and holds it steady in a position of 90° of flexion at the shoulder with the palm of the hand towards him. Active stabilisation of the thoracic spine is required, combined with activity in the oblique abdominal muscles (Fig. 4.27 a, b).

4.7 Position of the Arms

The position of the patient's arms is important. While carrying out activities involving the lower trunk and lower limbs, they should lie relaxed at his side. If the patient's affected arm becomes spastic and shows an associated reaction, the therapist should inhibit the hypertonus, place the arm at his side once again and ask him to make less effort when carrying out the activity. She may need to assist the movement more or reduce the amount of effort the patient makes by

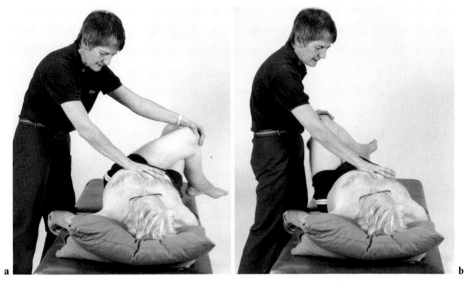

a   b

Fig. 4.25 a, b. Activating the oblique abdominals with the hemiplegic leg crossed over the sound leg (left hemiplegia). The crossed legs move rhythmically to the right and to the left. The therapist helps to stabilise the patient's thorax

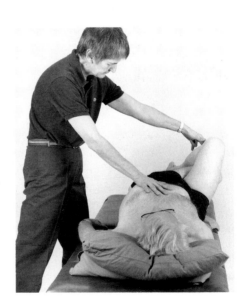

Fig. 4.26. With the sound leg crossed over the hemiplegic leg, the knees move to the left and right in approximately the rhythm of walking (left hemiplegia)

changing her verbal stimulus. It is contra-indicated to instruct the patient to hold his arms above his head to prevent flexion in the arm, as the rib cage will be elevated, the spine extended and the abdominals placed in a position of disadvantage (Fig. 4.28). In such a position the patient will almost certainly use to-

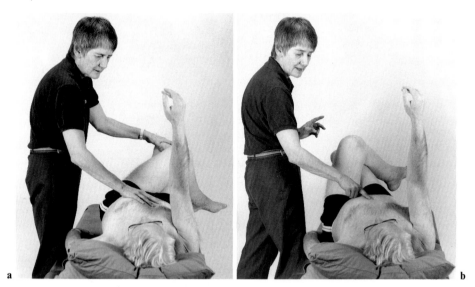

a   b

Fig. 4.27 a, b. With his sound arm held vertically in the air, the patient stabilises his thoracic spine actively as he moves his legs from side to side (left hemiplegia)

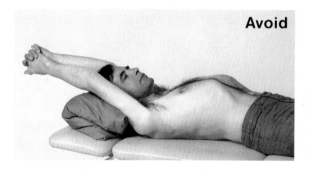

Avoid

Fig. 4.28. The patient should not hold his hands above his head when performing trunk activities as the rib cage will elevate and the spine extend (right hemiplegia)

tal extension of his trunk to stabilise his pelvis. Any associated reactions which occur should be regarded as a barometer or guide for the therapist, indicating that the activity is too difficult for the patient or that not enough assistance is being given him. Asking the patient to clasp his hands together and hold them over his head may disguise the fact that the hemiplegic arm is pulling into flexion. The hypertonus is still present, however, and the sound arm may suffer from the effort of prolonged holding. Some patients actually suffer from a supraspinatus tendinitis as a result. The painful condition can be very disabling as patients are dependent on the sound arm for carrying out all activities of daily living. It is important for the patient to learn to mentally inhibit the spastic reaction himself and to leave his arm lying at his side. The ultimate aim of low-

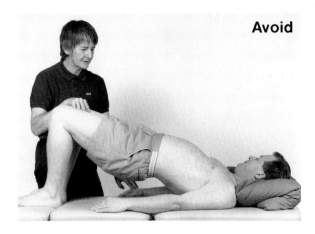

Avoid

Fig. 4.29. Bridging with too much extensor activity (right hemiplegia)

er trunk and leg activites is to enable the patient to walk more normally, and when walking, his arms need to remain relaxed for the arm swing.

4.8 Bridging, a Useful Activity for Regaining Selective Extension of the Hip Together with Abdominal Muscle Activity

The patient lies supine, with his head supported on a pillow and his arms relaxed at his sides. The therapist assists him as he flexes both legs at hip and knee. His feet are supported on the plinth so that his heels are not quite underneath his knees. When asked to raise his buttocks from the supporting surface, the patient will usually do so by extending his hips and arching his back in extension simultaneously, often pushing his head back on to the pillow as well (Fig. 4.29). To make the movement more selective, the therapist teaches the patient first to tilt his pelvis up in the front by contracting his lower abdominal muscles. She facilitates the correct movement by placing one hand over the patient's sound buttock and drawing the pelvis forwards and upwards. With her other hand she guides the umbilicus downwards and indicates the fulcrum around which the movement should take place (Fig. 4.30).

Holding his pelvis tipped up at the front, the patient lifts his seat from the plinth. The therapist asks him to lift his sound foot off the plinth and then place it back flat on the supporting surface while holding his seat in the air. He should lift and lower his foot repeatedly, in approximately the rhythm of normal walking. If not carefully instructed, the patient will lift his foot right up in the air to reinforce the inadequate hip extensors on the affected side. With the help of the therapist he tries to keep his pelvis level, i. e. not allowing it to drop down on the sound side (Fig. 4.31). Once he lifts his foot off the supporting surface, the leg becomes a "tentacle" and the pelvis must be held up by the muscles above, i. e. the abdominals. The "tentacle" effect is increased if the patient

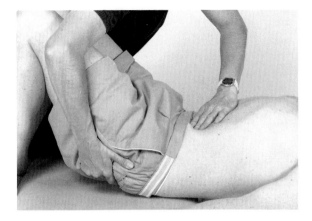

Fig. 4.30. Facilitating the correct position of the pelvis before bridging (right hemiplegia)

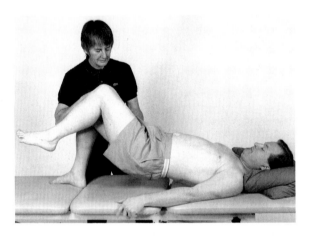

Fig. 4.31. Holding the pelvis level, the patient lifts his sound foot just off the plinth and then lowers it again (right hemiplegia)

holds his sound arm in the air at a right angle in relation to his trunk as he will not be able to press down on the surface to stabilise his trunk from below (Fig. 4.32a). The patient's affected arm remains at his side. If functional activity is present in the affected arm, however, he should hold both arms parallel to one another at 90° of shoulder flexion with the palms facing one another.

Additional activity and co-ordination are required when the patient lifts first one foot and then the other off the supporting surface without letting the pelvis sink down on either side. He should lift one foot after the other rhythmically in approximately the tempo of normal walking (Fig. 4.32b).

Many patients have difficulty holding the pelvis level, particularly when the sound foot is lifted from the plinth (Fig. 4.33a). The therapist can activate the appropriate oblique abdominal muscles by using carefully timed pressure tapping over their thoracic origin. The moment the patient lifts his sound foot off the plinth, she brings her cupped hand firmly and briskly down, "tapping" the muscles, increasing tone and stimulating activity. With the lumbrical muscles

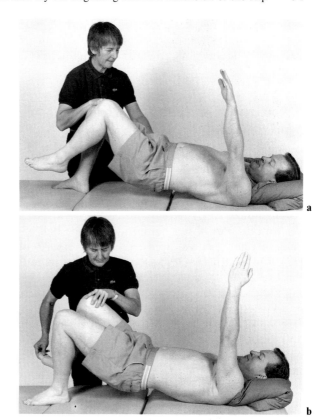

Fig. 4.32. a The patient holds his sound arm vertically above him as he lifts his sound foot. **b** Keeping the pelvis level when lifting the hemiplegic foot (right hemiplegia)

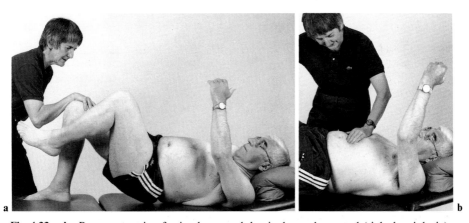

Fig. 4.33 a, b. Pressure tapping for inadequate abdominal muscle control (right hemiplegia). **a** The patient is unable to hold his pelvis level when he lifts the sound foot while bridging. **b** The therapist taps firmly over the origin of the external oblique abdominal muscles, at the exact moment when the sound foot is lifted

acting to hold her hand cupped and her fingers extended, the therapist taps with her hand placed so that it is in the direction of the muscle fibres, pointing diagonally downwards, towards the umbilicus (Fig. 4.33 b).

4.9 Actively Controlling the Hemiplegic Leg Through Its Range of Movement

The patient lies supine and the therapist moves his leg up into flexion at both the hip and the knee. With one of her hands she holds the patient's hemiplegic foot in dorsal flexion without supination and with the toes fully extended. She controls the foot by holding all the toes with her thumb and thenar eminence, yet with no part of her hand touching the ball of the patient's foot. The distal ends of her fingers apply counter-pressure on the dorsum of his foot (Fig. 4.34a). If necessary she uses her other hand to support the leg from below the knee. The therapist asks the patient to hold his leg actively in flexion without moving the hip into lateral rotation or abduction in the total flexion synergy. As he gains more control and holds the weight of his own leg actively (Fig. 4.34b), the patient follows the movement indicated by the therapist's hand and should eventually be able to maintain control until his leg is lying extended on the supporting surface. He should not resist the movement at all but follow instantaneously without his leg deviating in either inward or outward rotation.

The therapist moves the patient's sound leg in the same way, guiding it lightly, with one hand holding his toes (Fig. 4.35). The patient tries to keep his pelvis and lumbar spine flat on the plinth by tensing his abdominal muscles. The activity is progressed further by asking the patient to follow the movements

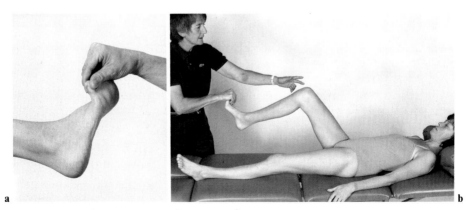

a   b

Fig. 4.34 a, b. Controlling the hemiplegic leg actively through range of movement (right hemiplegia). **a** The therapist supports the foot in dorsal flexion without supination, as a key point of control. **b** The patient holds her leg actively as the therapist moves it towards the supporting surface

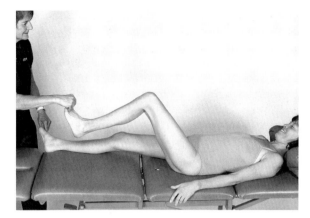

Fig. 4.35. Keeping the pelvis level while the sound leg is being guided through flexion and extension (right hemiplegia)

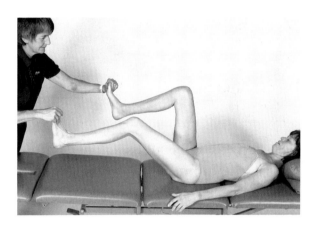

Fig. 4.36. The patient prevents her lumbar spine from becoming lordotic while both legs are following the movements actively (right hemiplegia)

indicated by the therapist's hands with both his legs. Both legs move independently and smoothly, which means that the patient cannot use his sound leg to stabilise his pelvis (Fig. 4.36). The ability to control the hemiplegic leg throughout its range of movement, particularly without its pushing into extension, is essential for the swing phase of walking. The activity is practised first in lying and later also in standing (see Chap. 8).

4.10 Conclusion

Selective activity of the hemiplegic arm and leg is dependent upon the patient's ability to control the trunk. Without a stable anchorage for the required muscles, movements of the limbs can only be performed in primitive, stereotyped mass patterns. Carefully preparing the required muscle activity for the various components of walking in lying will result in a more normal gait pattern later.

If the patient is encouraged to walk before he has regained sufficient control of his leg and trunk and their selective activity, he will do so by using typical sterotyped mass synergies (Perry 1969; Brunstrom 1970), with spasticity increasing as a result. Patients who have been walking abnormally for months or even years can still improve their gait pattern and regain confidence and ease of movement if the activities in lying are practised.

5 Moving Between Lying and Sitting

Moving from lying to sitting and from sitting to lying requires that the abdominal muscles move or hold the weight of the trunk against the pull of gravity or control the speed at which it moves. The head and trunk form a long lever, and their combined weight is considerable. The pull which gravity exerts on the trunk is far less when the body is nearer to the vertical than when almost in a horizontal lying position. Patients will have difficulty carrying out activities which require them to raise their head and trunk actively from the plinth, until they have regained tone and sufficient active control in their abdominal muscles. It is usually advisable, therefore, to start the movement with the patient sitting upright and move gradually further away from the more vertical position. Only when the patient is able to control the movement of his trunk with eccentric muscle activity right down to supine lying, will it be possible for him to start the movement from a horizontal position. The therapist should give the patient adequate support at all times as he will otherwise exert himself too much and distal spasticity will increase as a result. Care must be taken to ensure that the patient does not use compensatory movements, which he will do if the activity is too difficult for him.

5.1 Sitting Up over the Side of the Bed

Within a few days after the onset of hemiplegia, the patient should be helped to sit out of bed, either in an upright arm chair or a wheel chair. The way in which he is helped to sit up with his legs over the side of the bed and later to lie down again is very important. Left to his own devices, the patient will struggle to pull himself upright by using his sound hand. Associated reactions in the form of spasticity will result, usually with increased flexion in his arm and extension or flexion in his leg. From the very first, therefore, the patient should be taught to sit up in a normal sequence of movement which includes rotation of his trunk. He sits up over the hemiplegic side as follows:

- He lifts his hemiplegic leg up and over the side of the bed.
- His head and sound shoulder are lifted and rotated towards the hemiplegic side, with the arm coming forwards across his body until he can place his sound hand flat on the bed beside him.

- He brings his unaffected leg up and out of bed at the same time as he comes to the upright position, pushing down with his arm to assist the movement of his trunk if necessary.

Until he has learned to sit up correctly and without too much effort, the patient will need to be helped appropriately by the therapist or nurse.

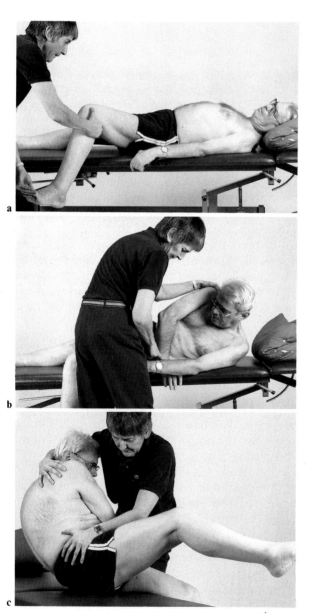

Fig. 5.1 a–c. Facilitation for sitting up over the side of the bed (left hemiplegia). **a** Bringing the hemiplegic leg actively over the side of the bed with help. **b** Flexing and rotating the trunk to place the sound hand on the opposite side of the bed for support. **c** Coming to sitting with the help of the assistant

5.1.1 Fully Supported

The assistant flexes the patient's hemiplegic leg and brings it over the side of the bed, one of her hands holding his foot in dorsal flexion, the other supporting the weight of his leg (Fig. 5.1 a).

She then helps him to lift his head and rotate his trunk towards her, which enables him to place his sound hand flat on the bed in front of him (Fig. 5.1 b).

With one arm around behind his shoulders, and her other hand pressing down on the side of his pelvis the assistant moves the patient to an upright position by transferring her weight sideways. The patient is asked to swing his sound leg out of bed at the same time, so that its weight helps to bring the trunk to a vertical position (Fig. 5.1 c). The movement is carried out slowly and carefully with clear instructions to the patient at each stage, so that he is able to help actively as much as he can.

5.1.2 Less Assistance

As soon as the patient is able to participate more actively and has regained some control of his trunk muscles, the assistant adjusts the amount of support accordingly. The patient brings his hemiplegic leg out of bed himself, while she ensures that his knee remains flexed. To help him to come to an upright position the assistant facilitates the movement by placing her hand on his sound shoulder, instead of having her arm around behind him. She presses down on his shoulder to facilitate the head righting to that side, as well as the necessary lateral flexion of the trunk (Fig. 5.2 a). Her other hand pushes down over the side of his pelvis to bring his sound buttock on to the supporting surface (Fig. 5.2 b).

5.1.3 No Support

The patient learns to sit up easily from lying on his own, finally without needing to push off from the bed with his sound hand (Fig. 5.3).

5.2 Lying Down from Sitting

To lie down from a sitting position with his legs over the side of the bed, the sequence of movement is similar to that used for coming upright, only in reverse order. The patient places his sound hand flat on the bed on the hemiplegic side to support some of the weight of the trunk. He lifts his sound leg and turns his body to lie down, bringing the hemiplegic shoulder well forwards. As he lies down, he lowers the sound leg to the bed and lifts his hemiplegic leg up as well.

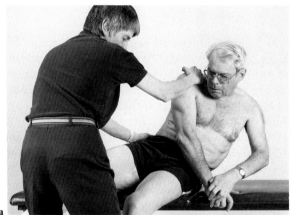

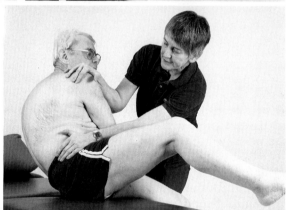

Fig. 5.2 a, b. Sitting up with facilitation from the shoulder and pelvis (left hemiplegia). **a** The assistant presses down on the shoulder to assist side flexion of the head and trunk. **b** The weight of the patient's leg helps him to sit up, as the assistant presses the side of the pelvis down towards the supporting surface

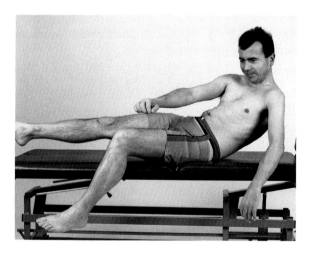

Fig. 5.3. The patient is able to sit up from lying by himself (left hemiplegia)

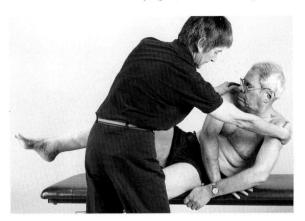

Fig. 5.4. Lying down from sitting. The assistant facilitates the movement by drawing the left shoulder forwards and supporting some of the weight of the trunk (left hemiplegia)

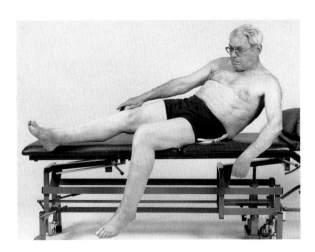

Fig. 5.5. Lying down on his own, without using the sound hand for support (left hemiplegia)

In the early stages, the patient will usually need to lie down completely so that his trunk is fully supported before he can flex the hemiplegic leg up on to the bed.

The assistant facilitates the movement of the patient's trunk by placing one hand behind his scapula to draw the hemiplegic shoulder forwards and support his weight as he lies down. Her other hand is placed in front of the patient's sound shoulder, guiding it backwards to assist the trunk rotation (Fig. 5.4). His sound hand leaves the supporting surface shortly before his head and shoulders come to rest on the bed. When the patient is lying supine, the assistant helps him to bring his hemiplegic leg up on to the bed, supporting its weight from beneath the thigh and keeping his foot in a neutral position. With her other hand the therapist holds his toes in extension. Later the patient should be able to lie down without needing to use his sound hand to support his weight (Fig. 5.5). It is beneficial to practise the different stages of the movement sequence separately, both those for sitting up and those for lying down again.

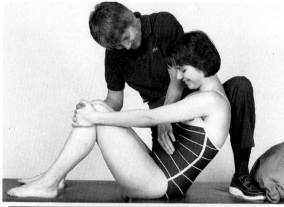

a

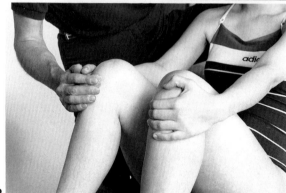

b

Fig. 5.6 a, b. Crook sitting. Adjusting the starting position (right hemiplegia). **a** The therapist supports the weight of the patient's trunk with her knee and the patient relaxes. **b** The patient's hands rest lightly on her knees, the therapist helping to hold the hemiplegic hand in place

5.3 Rocking in Crook Sitting

The patient often has difficulty flexing his lumbar spine. Over-activity of the extensors leads to a fixed lordotic position, and hypertonicity in the extensors of the leg increases as a result. The pelvis cannot move freely, and when walking, the patient flexes his whole trunk in order to bring his hemiplegic foot forwards. The lower abdominal muscles are unable to contract selectively if the lumbar spine is held in extension.

The patient sits on the plinth with his hips and knees flexed and his feet supported. One hand is placed around the front of each knee, the hemiplegic hand held in place by the therapist. The therapist will need to support the patient's trunk from behind with her leg. She places her foot on the plinth, and the patient can then lean against her leg confidently until his arms are relaxed and extended, and allow his lumbar spine to flex passively (Fig. 5.6a,b).

When the correct starting position has been achieved, the therapist moves her leg away, supporting the trunk with her arm around behind the patient's shoulders (Fig. 5.7a). He rocks backwards and forwards gently, using a selec-

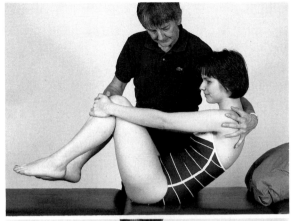

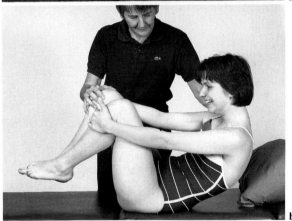

Fig. 5.7 a, b. Moving in crook sitting (right hemiplegia). **a** The patient rocks back and forth, using selective movement between her pelvis and lower trunk. **b** The therapist moves the patient gently from one side to the other to activate the trunk side flexors

tive movement between his pelvis and trunk. He is asked not to perform the activity by pulling with his arms, but to leave his elbows extended. As the patient's control improves he rocks further and further backwards.

When he can rock backwards and forwards easily, the therapist can move him towards one side to activate the side flexors of his trunk (Fig. 5.7 a).

5.4 Moving the Trunk in Long Sitting

Activities performed with the patient's extended legs supported on the plinth have the advantage that the pelvis is stabilised to a certain extent by the weight of the lower limbs. Selective activity between the trunk and the limbs is stimulated if the patient is asked to keep his legs flat on the plinth with his hips abducted and laterally rotated even though he is using the flexor muscles of his trunk.

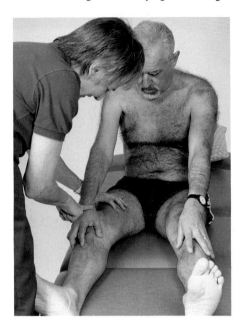

Fig. 5.8. Practising selective knee extension in long sitting. The patient's foot is kept in full dorsal flexion by the therapist's thigh, and his hands remains resting on his knees (right hemiplegia)

5.4.1 Long Sitting with Isolated Knee Extension

In long sitting the patient leaves both his hands resting lightly on his knees. He practises extending his knee selectively and then relaxing it again. The therapist maintains full dorsal flexion of his foot with her thigh (Fig. 5.8). If his hemiplegic hand remains stationary and does not slide towards him, the patient knows that he is not contracting his hip extensors when he tenses his knee. The active extension and relaxation is repeated rhythmically and can be alternated with contractions of the extensors of his other knee. The rhythm can be changed to make the activity more difficult, e. g. two contractions of his left knee followed by one of his right and vice versa. Isolated knee extension is very important for the patient in walking. If he cannot extend his knee selectively, it means that each time active knee extension takes place, his foot will plantarflex simultaneously. He will therefore not be able to bring his weight forwards adequately over his foot at the beginning of the stance phase as the resistance of his plantar flexors will oppose the movement. At the end of the swing phase the ball of his foot will reach the ground in front of him first. Because of the repeated plantar-flexor activity he may need to wear a calliper to hold his foot in dorsal flexion. The selective extension of the knee may need to be learned while the patient is lying down at first (Fig. 5.9). It is easier for him in a lying position because his hip is extended as well. It is essential that the therapist maintains full dorsal flexion of his ankle when he activates the knee extensors isometrically. He should be taught to carry out isolated extension of his sound knee accurately before attempting the activity on the hemiplegic side.

Selective knee extension is a prerequisite for walking without a support for

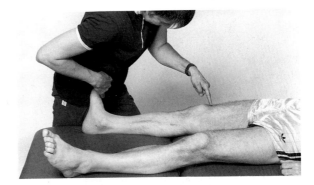

Fig. 5.9. Learning to extend the knee isometrically in lying at first. The foot remains inhibited in maximal dorsal flexion (right hemiplegia)

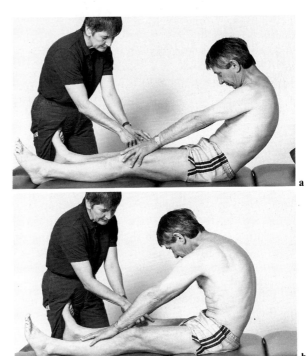

Fig. 5.10. a Keeping his knees and arms extended, the patient leans backwards, letting his hands slide along his thighs. **b** Moving forwards again, letting the hands glide towards his feet (right hemiplegia)

the foot. Regaining the activity will enable the patient to discard the calliper if he already has one.

5.4.2 Moving Towards Supine Lying

When the patient can extend his knee selectively in long sitting, he is asked to lean backwards and let his hands slide towards his hips while maintaining contact with his thighs. His elbows remain extended as his hands move towards his hips and then towards his feet again (Fig. 5.10a, b).

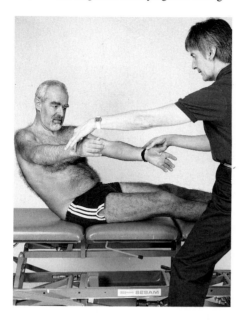

Fig. 5.11. Lying down from long sitting with rotation towards the hemiplegic side. The therapist holds the extended arms parallel to one another and shoulder width apart (right hemiplegia)

5.4.3 Lying Down with the Trunk Rotated

The patient in a long-sitting position turns towards the therapist who holds his hands lightly from above. She does not pull on his hands, but places them in the required position, with the patient holding them actively. His legs remain extended with the hips abducted (Fig. 5.11). The movement is performed first towards the hemiplegic side as it is less difficult for him to bring his sound shoulder forwards.

When he turns towards his sound side, the patient will have difficulty bringing the trunk on his hemiplegic side forwards and also keeping the leg extended as he does so. His hemiplegic leg will tend to flex as the trunk flexors on that side are acting (Fig. 5.12a). It may even pull up in the total pattern of flexion.

The therapist places one of her legs across the patient's thigh to hold the knee in extension, as he rotates his trunk towards her (Fig. 5.12b). He moves further and further towards the lying position and comes up to long sitting again each time.

When the therapist feels that the patient's leg is remaining flat on the bed and no longer pulling up against her leg, she asks him to maintain the extension actively (Fig. 5.12c).

When the patient can perform the movement accurately and keeps his leg extended without the help of the therapist, she stands at the side of the plinth and holds his hemiplegic foot in full dorsal flexion with her thigh. The patient keeps his arms extended and parallel to one another as he rotates his trunk and

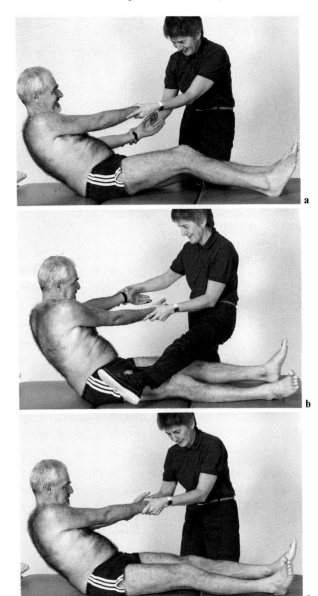

Fig. 5.12 a–c. Moving the trunk backwards in long sitting with rotation towards the sound side (right hemiplegia). **a** The patient has difficulty in bringing his affected shoulder forwards, and his hemiplegic leg tends to flex. **b** The therapist helps to keep the patient's leg in extension and holds his arms in the correct position. **c** The patient maintains the extension of his leg actively as he moves further and further towards lying and back up again

lies down, first to one side and then to the other. The therapist supports his hemiplegic arm in extension and guides his other arm into the correct position (Fig. 5.13 a, b).

Practising the activity reduces spasticity in the leg by moving the trunk proximally against the spastic limb distally, and the patient learns to extend his

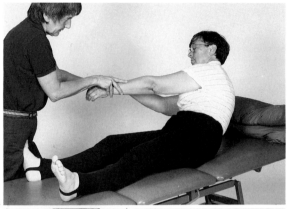

a

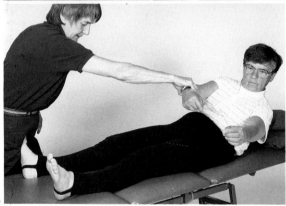

b

Fig. 5.13 a, b. Lying down from long sitting with trunk rotation. The therapist inhibits plantar flexion of the foot and corrects the position of the arms (right hemiplegia). **a** Rotating to the hemiplegic side. **b** Rotating to the sound side

leg selectively. Active control of the trunk, particularly the activity of the oblique abdominal muscles, is improved considerably.

5.5 Conclusion

It is important for the patient to be able to get out of his bed alone and to lie down when he so wishes without the help of another person. The muscle activity which is stimulated by moving between lying and sitting will not only enable him to sit up and lie down independently, but will also improve his ability to perform other activities. Normal balance reactions will be made possible, as will his ability to climb stairs, get in and out of the bath, etc. The activities described in the chapter should be practised thoroughly during treatment and not only once a day when the patient is being assisted to sit up out of bed.

6 Activities in Sitting

Activities practised with the patient sitting provide a good opportunity for stimulating the muscles controlling the trunk. Moving the patient, or asking him to move sideways, forwards or backwards will mean that his body becomes the "tentacle" as described in Chap. 2. The muscles on the uppermost side of the trunk in relation to the pull of gravity will be activated, either to move the body actively against gravity, to hold it in a position or to control the speed of movement in the direction of gravity.

6.1 Sitting with Both Legs over the Side of the Plinth

Many of the following activities can also be performed with the patient sitting on his bed, on a chair or on a bench in the occupational therapy department. It is, however, easier for the patient at first if his feet are not supported. With his feet on the floor, he will try to use his sound foot to help him to carry out the movement and use compensatory muscles as a result. It is also difficult for the therapist to control unwanted associated reactions in his hemiplegic foot, while at the same time facilitating the correct movements of the trunk. However, in our daily lives we usually perform functional activities when sitting with our feet on the floor, and once the patient has learned an activity, it should also be carried out in the normal sitting position.

6.1.2 Selective Flexion and Extension of the Lower Trunk

Before practising other activities in sitting, it is important that the patient learns to correct his posture. Stabilisation of the thoracic spine is a prerequisite for normal walking as well as for selective skilled movements of the arms.

Left to his own devices the patient will sit with his hips in too much extension and his thoracic spine kyphotic. He will need to correct the position of his pelvis before being able to achieve an upright posture.

The therapist stands in front of the patient and places one of her hands over his hemiplegic shoulder, to prevent it from pulling back. With her other hand over his lumbar spine she helps him to extend his spine and flex his hips

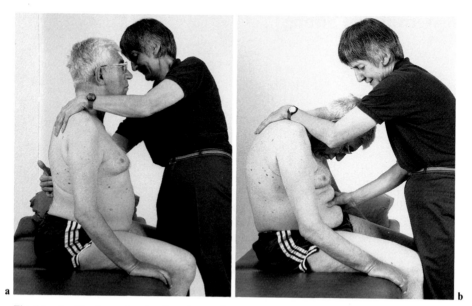

Fig. 6.1 a, b. Flexing and extending the trunk to correct the position of the pelvis (right hemiplegia). **a** Extension. **b** Flexion

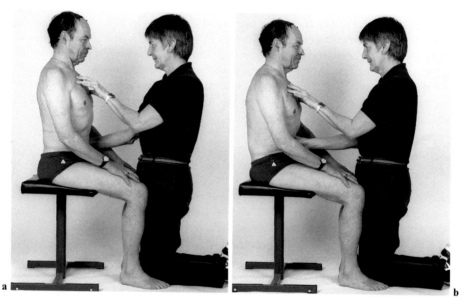

Fig. 6.2 a, b. Selective movement of the lower trunk with stabilisation of the thoracic spine (right hemiplegia). **a** Extension. **b** Flexion

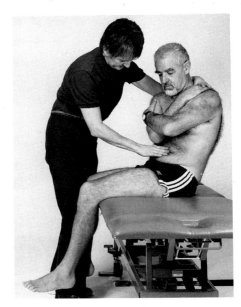

Fig. 6.3. Active flexion and rotation of the trunk. The patient uses his sound hand to draw the opposite shoulder forwards (right hemiplegia)

(Fig. 6.1a). Keeping her hand on his affected shoulder she then instructs the patient to flex his whole spine and uses her other hand to assist his abdomen to sink backwards (Fig. 6.1b). His neck flexes as well. When he can straighten and round his back in a total pattern, the movement can be practised more and more selectively.

The therapist asks the patient to keep his head and shoulders erect and to flex and extend only his lower back. She indicates that the movement should take place only below the level of his umbilicus.

As the patient's ability to stabilise his thoracic spine while flexing and extending his lumbar spine increases, he can practise the movement while sitting on a chair or stool with his feet on the ground (Fig. 6.2a,b).

6.1.3 Trunk Rotation with Flexion

The patient sits upright and the therapist helps him to place his hemiplegic hand on his opposite shoulder. With his sound hand holding the affected upper arm he helps to draw the scapula forwards as the therapist moves his trunk backwards, behind his centre of gravity (Fig. 6.3). She puts her arm round behind him and with her fingers over his keeps his hand in place while at the same time pressing his hemiplegic shoulder forwards and downwards with her arm. With her other hand she brings his ribs down and together in the middle and indicates to the patient where the muscle activity should take place. As a result the patient's elbow should move in the direction of his contralateral hip.

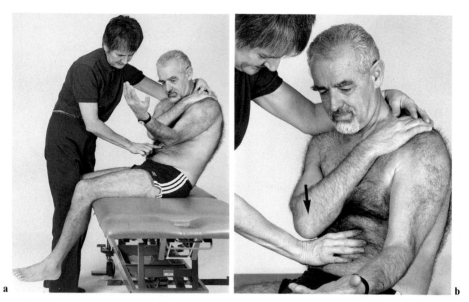

Fig. 6.4 a, b. Flexion/rotation of the trunk against gravity (right hemiplegia). **a** The patient holds his sound arm forwards with adduction and lateral rotation of the shoulder. His hemiplegic hand stays in position with the fingers relaxed. **b** The therapist facilitates the correct movement of the hemiplegic shoulder, forwards, and down towards the contralateral hip

The patient repeats the movement with the sound arm held in a position of flexion, adduction with outward rotation of the shoulder with elbow flexion (Fig. 6.4a, b). The position of the sound arm is important as the patient will otherwise automatically extend it behind him and use unilateral extensor activity of his trunk for the rotation, and not the desired abdominal activity. Care must be taken that the lumbar spine is flexed and does not extend over-actively. The patient's legs should remain hanging over the side of the plinth and not pull up into hip flexion. The activity is performed with progressively less help from the therapist until the patient can hold his arm in place alone and without effort (Fig. 6.5).

It can also be practised with both feet remaining on the floor. At first there is often resistance to flexing the affected elbow when the shoulder is protracted and adducted. The rotation of the trunk inhibits the extensor hypertonus in the arm, and once no resistance to flexion is felt, the patient can be asked to flex his elbow actively with help and replace his hand on his shoulder, when the therapist has moved it increasingly further away (Fig. 6.6. a, b). The elbow flexion should be carried out selectively without the scapula retracting.

Many functional activities such as eating, washing and grooming require flexion of the arm in front of the body, and learning to perform the movement selectively prepares the way for the patient to use his hemiplegic hand for such activities in his daily life.

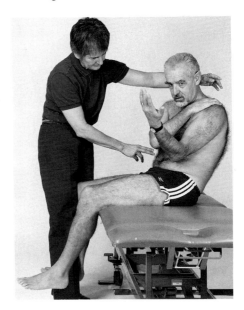

Fig. 6.5. Maintaining the position actively without assistance (right hemiplegia)

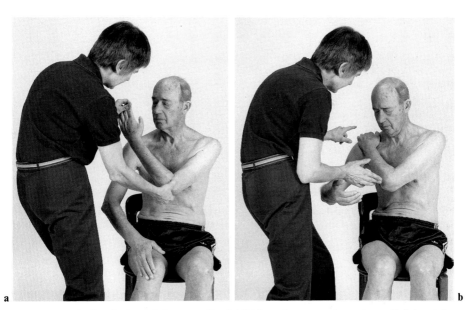

Fig. 6.6 a, b. Active flexion of the arm after inhibition of extensor hypertonus (left hemiplegia). **a** The therapist moves the patient's hand away from his shoulder, increasing the distance gradually each time. **b** The patient replaces his hand actively by flexing his elbow without retraction of the affected scapula

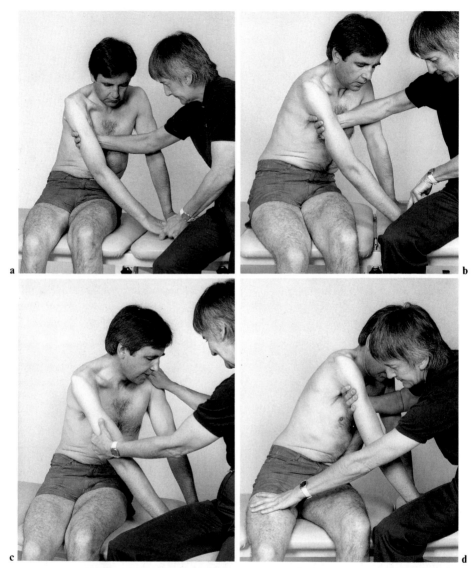

Fig. 6.7 a–d. Rotation of the trunk towards the sound side (right hemiplegia). **a** Placing the hemiplegic hand flat on the plinth. **b** Assisting flexion of the upper trunk and protraction of the shoulder. **c** Guiding the sound shoulder back while holding the hemiplegic arm in position. **b** Adjusting the position of the patient's hip and pelvis

Fig. 6.8 a, b. Flexion/rotation of the trunk with both arms supported on the sound side (right hemiplegia). **a** The therapist prevents adduction of the right hip and assists elbow extension. **b** Using a lumbrical grip to extend the elbow and give pressure through the heel of the patient's hand

6.2 Rotation of the Trunk with Both Arms Supported on the Same Side

6.2.1 Rotating Towards the Sound Side

With his sound hand resting on the plinth beside him, the patient turns towards that side, and the therapist helps him to place his hemiplegic hand on the plinth as well, parallel to the other hand. Due to the inability to rotate the hemiplegic side forwards, his arm will seem to be too short, and his hand may not reach the plinth. Sitting beside the patient, the therapist uses one of her hands to hold his upper arm near the shoulder and draw it forwards. With the back of her wrist she applies counter-pressure to the patient's sternum to help him flex his thoracic spine and protract his scapula (Fig. 6.7 a). Her other hand guides his hand flat onto the surface of the plinth with the fingers and thumb lying extended.

Because she needs her hand to correct other parts of the patient's body, she holds his hand on the plinth with her thigh, resting her leg gently on his extended hand (Fig. 6.7 b). The patient will usually move his hips to compensate for the insufficient trunk rotation, the hemiplegic hip being brought forward and adducted. The therapist should first correct the position of the shoulders and trunk before sorting out the position of his pelvis and hemiplegic leg.

Most patients will make too much effort with their sound arm, holding that shoulder forwards actively, and so preventing the trunk rotation. With her freed hand the therapist guides the patient's sound shoulder backwards and facilitates the trunk rotation (Fig. 6.7 c).

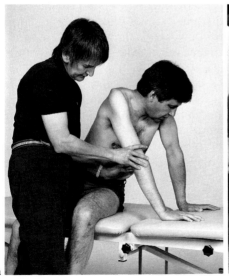
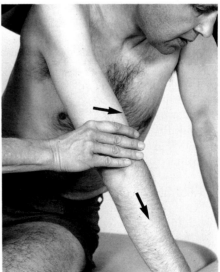

a   b

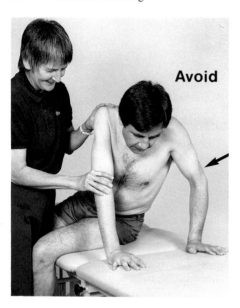

Fig. 6.9. The patient should not flex the sound elbow to compensate for lack of trunk rotation (right hemiplegia)

Once both shoulders are in the correct position the therapist places one hand on the patient's thigh to hold his hemiplegic leg in more abduction and keep his seat flat on the plinth (Fig. 6.7 d).

When the hemiplegic shoulder is no longer pulling backwards, and the flexor spasticity in the hand has been reduced, the therapist changes her position. She stands in front of the patient and maintains the abducted position of his hemiplegic leg with her leg. She uses one of her hands to assist full extension of the elbow on his affected side and at the same time to keep the shoulder forwards. Her hand over the condyles of the humerus not only gives pressure in the direction of elbow extension, but also downwards through the heel of the patient's hand (Fig. 6.8 a,b). The back of her other hand over his lower ribs guides the trunk into flexion.

The patient is instructed to relax and just remain in this position without exertion and then to move gently, shifting his weight first over one hand and then over the other. He experiences the weight going through the lateral border of the palm of his hand and, as he moves towards the other side, the pressure changing to its medial border. The weight shifting from one side of his hand to the other releases the flexor spasticity amazingly. Because only one of her hands is required to maintain the position of the hemiplegic arm, the therapist can use her other hand to correct compensatory evasive movements, e. g. the patient will often automatically flex his sound elbow if his trunk does not rotate sufficiently (Fig. 6.9), which the therapist may not notice.

Another common compensatory mechanism is extension of the trunk (Fig. 6.10 a). The therapist must frequently guide his thorax back into flexion using the dorsum of her free hand (Fig. 6.10 b).

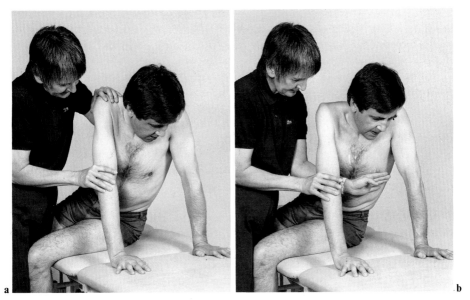

Fig. 6.10 a, b. Avoiding compensatory trunk extension. **a** With the trunk extended the rotation takes place in the hips. **b** The therapist guides the trunk into flexion with the back of her hand (right hemiplegia)

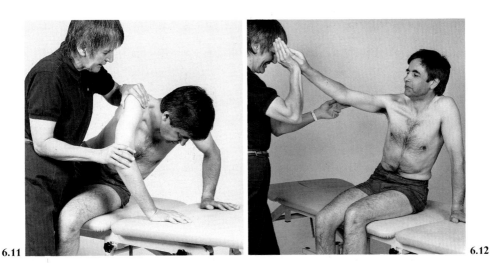

Fig. 6.11. The patient flexes his elbows and brings his head down towards the plinth, his nose directly over the midpoint between his hands (right hemiplegia)

Fig. 6.12. Active extension of the elbow with the hemiplegic shoulder kept forward (right hemiplegia)

The patient is asked to flex both of his elbows and move his nose towards the plinth. The sound elbow must move in a direction parallel to that of the affected elbow. The patient moves his head down only as far as is possible without his buttock leaving the plinth (Fig. 6.11).

After the trunk rotation and reduction of spasticity in the upper limb, the patient is asked to hold his extended arm forwards, with his hand against that of the therapist without overexertion. By keeping the patient's hand forward, as the therapist gives light pressure through the heel of his hand, the oblique abdominal muscles are activated (Fig. 6.12).

6.2.2 Rotating Towards the Hemiplegic Side

The therapist guides the patient's hemiplegic arm around to the other side and places his hand flat on the plinth beside him at about the level of his trochanter. While she supports the patient's elbow in extension he brings his sound hand forwards and places it in line with his other hand, and shoulder width apart. The therapist's other hand brings his hemiplegic shoulder backwards, and her forearm over his scapula draws it into the correct position (Fig. 6.13). She needs to help considerably to achieve the position because the patient, in his efforts to extend his arm, will be using the synergistic action of protraction with adduction of the arm. Such activity on the hemiplegic side prevents trunk rotation. The therapist asks the patient to bring his nose down towards the plinth, in the middle of the space between his hands. She should notice if his sound elbow, on the side away from her, is moving in the right direction. It should be moving along a line parallel to that of the hemiplegic elbow. Often, due to too little trunk rotation, the sound elbow moves towards the unaffected

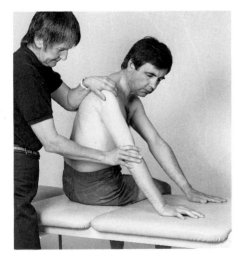

Fig. 6.13. Flexion/rotation of the trunk with both hands supported on the hemiplegic side. The therapist draws the shoulder back and assists elbow extension (right hemiplegia)

side instead (Fig. 6.14a). The therapist uses her hand to indicate the optimal movement direction (Fig. 6.14b), but once the patient understands what is expected of him, she will need to use her hand once again to support the shoulder and scapula on the affected side (Fig. 6.14c).

As the elbows flex, the weight moves over to the lateral border of the palm of the hand, and as they extend, it returns to the medial border.

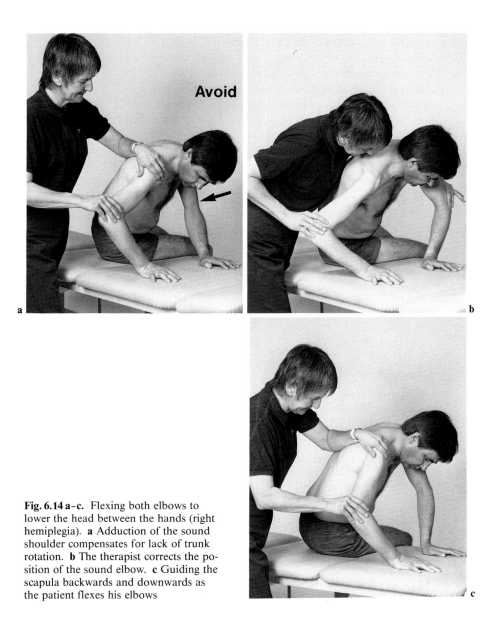

Fig. 6.14 a–c. Flexing both elbows to lower the head between the hands (right hemiplegia). **a** Adduction of the sound shoulder compensates for lack of trunk rotation. **b** The therapist corrects the position of the sound elbow. **c** Guiding the scapula backwards and downwards as the patient flexes his elbows

6.3 Active Movements of the Hemiplegic Arm Following the Inhibition of Spasticity

With spasticity greatly reduced by the activities involving trunk rotation and weight shifting over the extended arms, the patient can be asked to move his hemiplegic arm actively and selectively. Actual objects to hold, to cut, to drink and to move will facilitate normal movement. The activity and the amount of assistance the therapist gives depends on the degree of active function which the patient has regained (Davies 1985). Most patients will have difficulties re-gaining active supination of the arm while the hand is holding something. The hypertonus in the pronators should first be inhibited by proximal movement and then assisted active movements practised.

The patient holds a thick wooden pole in both his hands. The hands should be shoulder width apart. The therapist stands beside him with one of her feet on a stool in front of him, and he supports his elbows on her knee. It is impor-tant that his elbows or upper arms are supported as his hemiplegic shoulder could otherwise be traumatised (Fig. 6.15a). The therapist supports his hemi-plegic hand in such a way that the wrist remains dorsiflexed although he is grasping the pole.

The therapist then uses her other hand to help the patient flex his spine, in-dicating the lower abdomen. The patient usually flexes the thoracic spine, but has difficulty in flexing the lumbar region (Fig. 6.15b).

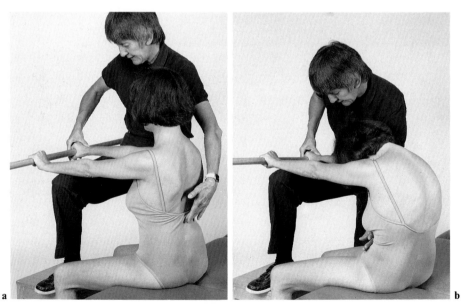

Fig. 6.15 a, b. Moving the trunk while holding a pole in both hands (right hemiplegia). **a** Trunk extension with the patient's elbows supported. **b** The therapist assists trunk flexion

After flexing and extending the trunk proximally against the distal spasticity in the arms, the hypertonus is reduced, and the therapist helps the patient to supinate his arms and grasp the pole with both hands, once more at shoulder width from one another (Fig. 6.16). In supination, he will probably have difficulty maintaining flexion of the fingers, and the therapist will need to hold his fingers and his thumb around the pole and maintain dorsal flexion of the wrist.

The patient flexes and extends his trunk while his hands remain motionless, with his elbows still supported on the therapist's thigh. With one of her hands the therapist adjusts the location of the movement, either to prevent hypermo-

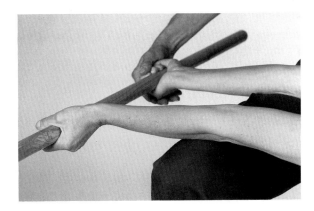

Fig. 6.16. Holding the pole with supination of the forearm (right hemiplegia)

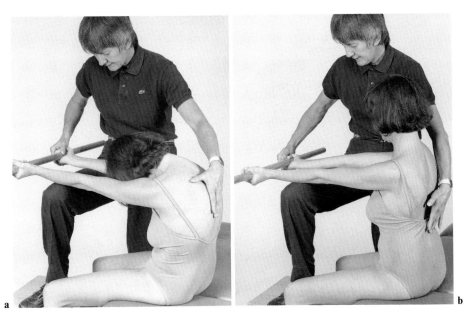

a

b

Fig. 6.17 a, b. Moving the trunk proximally against the distal spasticity in the arm (right hemiplegia). **a** Flexion. **b** Extension

bility of one part (Fig. 6.17a) or to encourage further range of movement at another (Fig. 6.17b).

When the therapist feels that the patient's fingers and wrist are remaining in the correct position on the pole, she takes her hands slowly away. When his hand remains in place, the patient is asked to remove his sound hand from the pole and let it rest on his knee (Fig. 6.18).

The patient then tries to hold the pole horizontally with his hemiplegic hand, i.e. without allowing any pronation. He can also turn it slightly towards pronation and then back into supination again.

With his elbow still supported on the therapist's thigh, he brings the pole towards his head, keeping it parallel to his trunk (Fig. 6.19a–c).

If his elbows are not supported by the therapist's thigh, the movement becomes more difficult as the patient must stabilise his scapula actively. He learns to move the pole towards his head and away again without his scapulae winging (Fig. 6.20a). Gradually he learns to maintain the position of the scapula on the hemiplegic side even when he brings the sound hand away from the pole (Fig. 6.20b).

6.4 Weight Transference Sideways

To move or be moved sideways in sitting requires balance reactions which are dependent upon much selective trunk activity, particularly lateral flexion combined with extension of both the thoracic and the lumbar spine. Lateral flexion of the trunk against gravity requires considerable activity of the abdominal

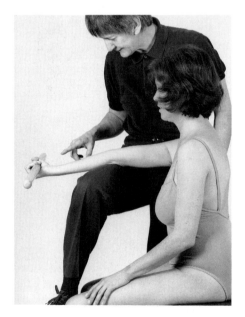

Fig. 6.18. Holding the pole with the forearm supinated after inhibition of spasticity (right hemiplegia)

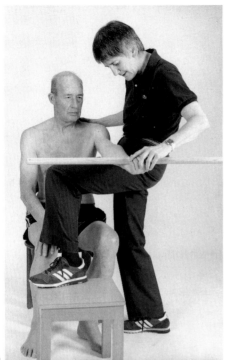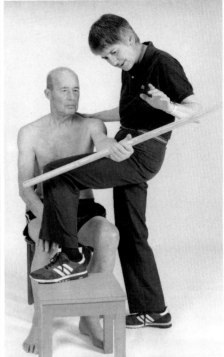

a

b

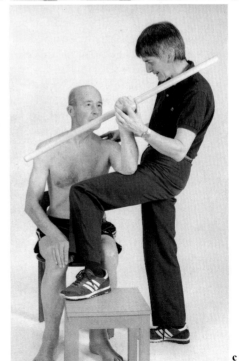

Fig. 6.19 a–c. Holding the pole and moving the arm actively (left hemiplegia).
a The patient's elbow is supported on the therapist's thigh. **b** Selective elbow flexion. **c** Moving the pole with active pro- and supination

c

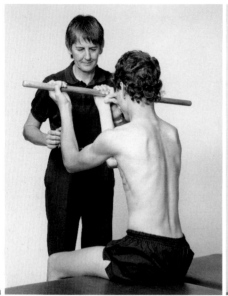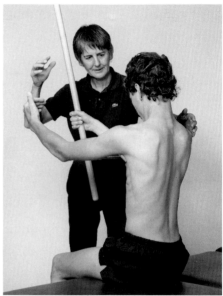

Fig. 6.20 a, b. Stabilising the scapula actively while moving the pole (right hemiplegia) **a** with both hands and **b** with the hemiplegic hand alone

muscles (Flint and Gudgell 1965), particularly a vigorous contraction of the external obliques (Campbell and Green 1953). The balance reactions are necessary for functional activities carried out in a sitting position, such as putting on socks and shoes. The selective muscle activity demanded by the correct execution of the balance reactions is essential for normal gait.

Once the patient is able to move freely and without fear over both sides, with facilitation from the therapist, the reactions should be refined and practised more exactly with less and less support, until they take place automatically even at speed and with unexpected changes in direction.

6.4.1 Moving Towards the Hemiplegic Side

Even the well-trained patient will tend to maintain his balance through an evasive movement which requires less selective activity (Fig. 6.21 a,b). The head rights, the trunk flexes laterally and the sound arm and leg lift in abduction and extension. However, the lateral flexion of the trunk is not selective. The patient sinks backwards on the supporting side and flexes the whole trunk simultaneously. He is unable to extend the thoracic and lumbar spine and elevates the sound shoulder to compensate for the inadequate extension. The sound leg appears to be too far in abduction, and the side of the pelvis is back on that side. With careful instruction and practising the movement with the help of the therapist, the correct reactions can be trained (Fig. 6.22 a,b).

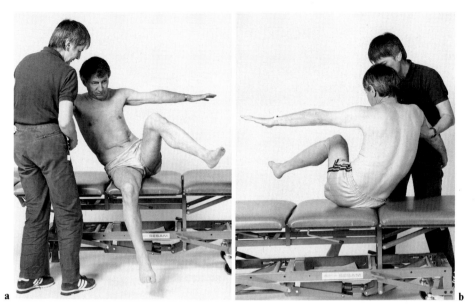

Fig. 6.21 a, b. Balance reactions with the weight transferred over the hemiplegic side (right hemiplegia). **a** Anterior view: the trunk movement is not selective and the sound leg abducts too much. **b** Posterior view: the spine flexes in a total pattern

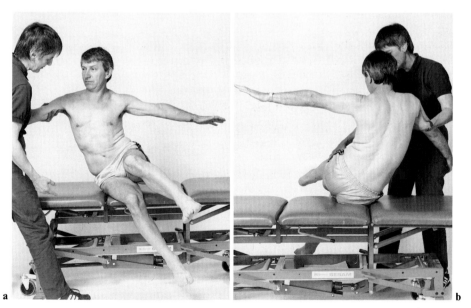

Fig. 6.22 a, b. Balance reactions with the weight transferred towards the hemiplegic side (right hemiplegia). **a** With selective trunk activity the leg reacts normally. **b** Side flexion occurs without total flexion of the spine

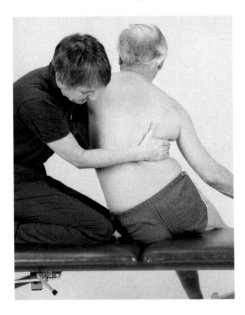

Fig. 6.23. Passive mobilisation for lateral flexion of the lumbar spine (left hemiplegia)

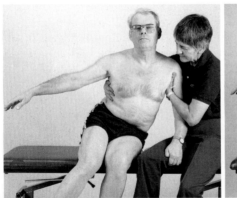
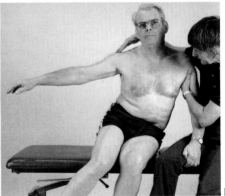

a

b

Fig. 6.24 a, b. Facilitating active side flexion of the trunk with the weight shifted towards the hemiplegic side (left hemiplegia). **a** The therapist assists shortening of the sound side and lengthening of the hemiplegic side. **b** Correcting compensatory elevation of the shoulder girdle on the sound side

6.4.1.1 A Progressive Sequence to Teach the Correct Movement

The therapist kneels on the bed beside the patient and with one arm behind and the other in front of him, clasps her hands around him at about the level of his lower ribs on his other side. She asks the patient to allow her to move him without any resistance, but without his trying to help her actively. She moves

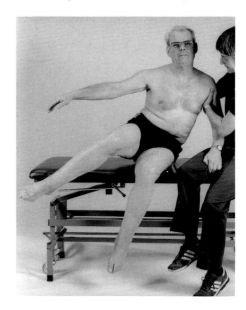

Fig. 6.25. Maintaining trunk extension with side flexion when the sound leg is lifted (left hemiplegia)

his trunk sideways, rhythmically using her hands to obtain lateral flexion of the lumbar spine passively while her arms keep his trunk extended. With her head behind the patient, the therapist is able to observe the lumbar region and see whether the side flexion is really taking place in his lumbar spine (Fig. 6.23).

When passive side flexion is occurring freely, the therapist sits beside the patient and draws his weight towards her over his hemiplegic side. Her hand in his axilla helps the side to lengthen in a normal way, and with her other arm behind him and her hand in his waist on the sound side, she indicates the required shortening (Fig. 6.24a).

Many patients will elevate their sound shoulder in an attempt to compensate for the inadequate hip extension required on the supporting hemiplegic side. Raising the shoulder girdle in this way prevents trunk side flexion. The therapist uses her hand to indicate to the patient that his shoulder should move downwards instead (Fig. 6.24b).

When he can move far enough over towards the hemiplegic side, the therapist asks the patient to lift his sound leg in the air (Fig. 6.25). Once the patient can move easily over his hemiplegic side with only minimal assistance from the therapist, she can then stand in front of him. If his arm does not function actively she supports it against the side of her body, holding his upper arm to protect his shoulder and to help elongate the side (Fig. 6.26a,b). With her other hand she helps the patient lift his sound leg into the correct position, giving only as much support as he requires (Fig. 6.27).

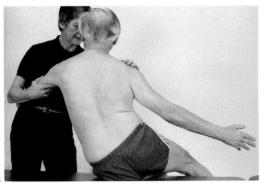
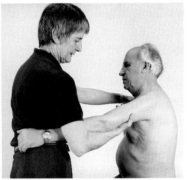

a   b

Fig. 6.26 a, b. Facilitating balance reactions with the weight shifted over the hemiplegic side (left hemiplegia). **a** The therapist supports the affected arm and guides the sound shoulder downwards. **b** The hemiplegic arm is supported from below to protect the shoulder

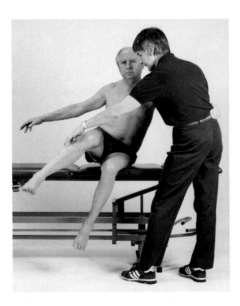

Fig. 6.27. Correcting the reaction of the sound leg (left hemiplegia)

6.4.2 Moving Towards the Sound Side

The patient has great difficulty in transferring his weight over the sound side. The normal balance reactions involve lateral flexion of the neck and trunk on the hemiplegic side and flexion/abduction of the extending hemiplegic leg. All these components are dependent upon considerable abdominal muscle activity to stabilise both thorax and pelvis and also to flex the side of the trunk. The patient is usually not able to abduct his extended leg to act as a counter-weight.

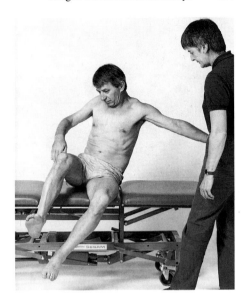

Fig. 6.28. Abnormal balance reactions due to inadequate selective trunk activity when the weight is transferred towards the sound side (right hemiplegia)

The hemiplegic shoulder elevates and the trunk does not shorten on that side. If his leg can be lifted at all, it flexes in a total mass pattern, with the pelvis pulling back. The knee cannot be extended selectively, and the foot supinates with dorsal flexion (Fig. 6.28).

6.4.2.1 A Progressive Sequence to Teach the Correct Movement

If the patient cannot actively shorten the side of his trunk (Fig. 6.29), the therapist kneels beside him on his sound side, with his arm resting across her shoulder. She places one of her arms in front of him and the other behind and clasps her hands over his lower ribs on the hemiplegic side. Asking the patient to allow the movement to occur without any resistance she moves him rhythmically towards her, using her shoulder under his arm to elongate the sound side and her hands to shorten the hemiplegic side (Fig. 6.30). Once again, she can observe his lumbar spine as she does so to see if side flexion is taking place.

When the passive side flexion is taking place freely, the therapist sits beside the patient on his hemiplegic side and asks him to move away from her. With one of her hands on top of his hemiplegic shoulder, she presses down to facilitate the head righting reaction. With her other hand she uses the web between her thumb and index finger to stimulate the side flexion of his trunk. She must also remind the patient to keep his spine extended (Fig. 6.31). The movement is practised without the patient being asked to lift his hemiplegic leg consciously from the plinth. When he can move his trunk without help, or with only slight assistance, the therapist can facilitate the reaction of his leg.

If he has difficulty in letting his hemiplegic leg react correctly and selectively, the therapist sits in front of him on a stool which is lower than the plinth

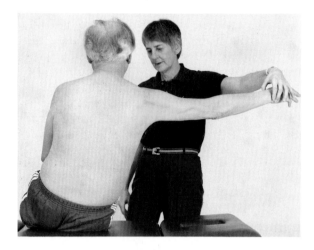

Fig. 6.29. Inadequate side flexion of the trunk when the weight is shifted to the sound side (left hemiplegia)

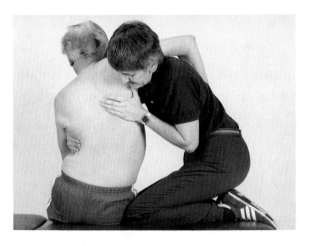

Fig. 6.30. Mobilising lateral flexion of the trunk in preparation for active shortening (left hemiplegia)

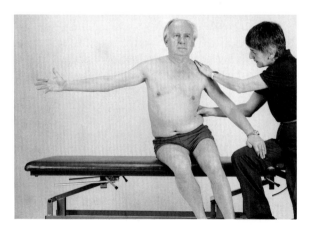

Fig. 6.31. Facilitating active side flexion of the trunk with the weight shifted to the sound side (left hemiplegia)

and supports his leg on her knee. The patient transfers his weight to the sound side and the therapist uses one of her hands placed over his shoulder to assist the shortening of the side of his trunk. With her other hand she holds his hemiplegic leg extended and relaxed on her knee. With one of her legs she ensures adduction and outward rotation of his sound leg (Fig. 6.32 a). The patient returns to a sitting position and then moves repeatedly over towards his sound side and back again, consciously relaxing his supported leg until the hypertonus is reduced. The therapist keeps his knee in extension, inhibits adduction of the leg, and with her other hand prevents the foot from pulling into supination as the patient moves proximally against the distal spasticity. When she feels that the knee and foot are no longer pulling into flexion, she lifts the leg up when the patient has transferred his weight well over to the sound side and asks him to leave it in the air. She supports some of its weight, just sufficient to avoid his having to use too much effort to hold his leg in the air in the correct position (Fig. 6.32 b).

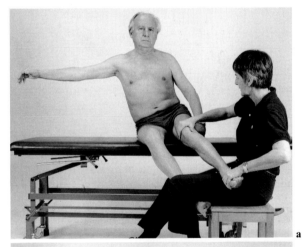

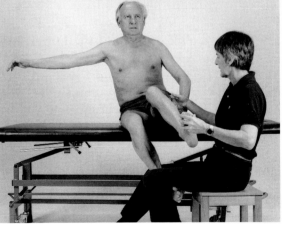

Fig. 6.32 a, b. Retraining balance reactions in the hemiplegic leg (left hemiplegia). **a** The therapist supports the weight of the leg and inhibits the total pattern of flexion. **b** She guides the leg into the correct position

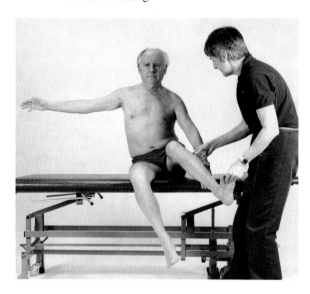

Fig. 6.33. Facilitating the leg reaction from the foot with only minimal assistance (left hemiplegia)

Finally, as the patient transfers his weight over the sound side correctly and quite alone, the therapist stands in front of him and facilitates the leg reaction from the foot, giving only minimal assistance (Fig. 6.33).

Quick changes in direction, with automatic balance reactions are important during the activities of daily life. Many patients will demonstrate normal reactions in a therapeutic situation when they are cued by the therapist and her position, but will fail to react correctly if the situation is changed. The patient should eventually be able to react quickly and automatically with the therapist standing behind him, signalling unexpected changes in direction with her hands, and not always by drawing his arm sideways while standing at his side (Fig. 6.34a, b).

6.5 Selective Side Flexion of the Lower Trunk

The patient sits with one leg crossed over the other with his feet not touching the floor at first. With his weight on the side of the leg underneath he lifts the buttock on the opposite side off the supporting surface and lowers it again repeatedly. His spine remains extended and his shoulders on one level throughout the activity, so that the movement takes place selectively in the lumbar spine. The activity is practised to both sides, with the appropriate leg being crossed over the other.

The therapist stands in front of the patient and places one of her hands on his thoracic spine, her arm over the top of his shoulder on the side of the supporting leg. As he lifts his buttock she can help him to stabilise his thoracic

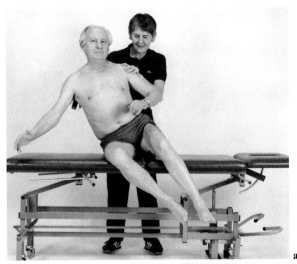

a

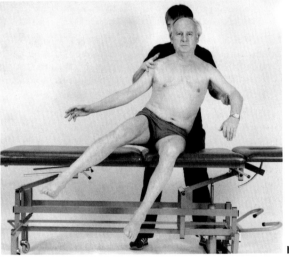

b

Fig. 6.34 a, b. Reacting automatically to quick unexpected changes in direction (left hemiplegia). **a** Weight transference to the sound side. **b** Weight transference to the hemiplegic side

spine and should his head not right to the vertical, she can guide it with her arm, asking him at the same time to move his head away from her forearm (Fig. 6.35 a, b). The therapist places her other hand beneath the patient's buttock on the opposite side and helps him to raise it easily and rhythmically off the plinth. He can also be asked to hold the position with his buttock off the plinth.

The starting position for the activity facilitates selective side flexion of the lower trunk, with weight over the underneath leg because the heavy lever of the other leg is supported from below and is not dependent upon the muscles above to lift its weight. The action of crossing one leg over the other in itself incorporates an automatic transference of weight towards the side of the under-

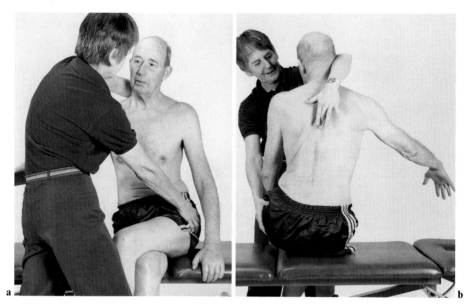

Fig. 6.35 a, b. Selective side flexion of the lower trunk with one leg crossed over the other (left hemiplegia). **a** With the weight on the side of the underneath leg, the patient lifts and lowers the buttock on the opposite side. **b** The therapist facilitates the lifting movement and helps to stabilise the thoracic spine with her other hand

neath leg. Should the patient have difficulty in keeping his hemiplegic leg crossed over the other, due to spastic retraction of the side of his pelvis or extensor hypertonus in his knee, the therapist holds the limb in place with her legs while using her hands to assist the correct movement of the trunk. As the activity is repeated, spasticity in the leg is inhibited by the proximal movement of the trunk. The therapist can reduce the amount of support given to keep the leg in place and also to stabilise the thorax (Fig. 6.36). The patient later practises the movement with the foot on the weight-bearing side flat on the floor (Fig. 6.37 a, b).

6.6 Active Side Flexion of the Trunk Against Gravity

The patient leans towards his sound side and supports his weight on his elbow. He then returns to an upright sitting position without using his sound arm to push off from the plinth, holding it instead with the elbow in 90° of flexion. The muscles on the uppermost side of the trunk are activated and the head rights towards the hemiplegic side.

The therapist stands in front of the patient and guides his sound elbow down onto the plinth, if necessary supporting his weight with her other arm

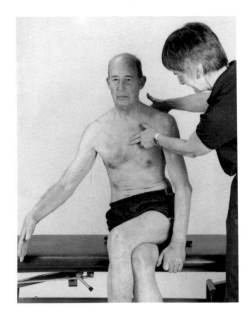

Fig. 6.36. Selective lateral flexion of the lumber spine with a little help in stabilising the thorax (left hemiplegia)

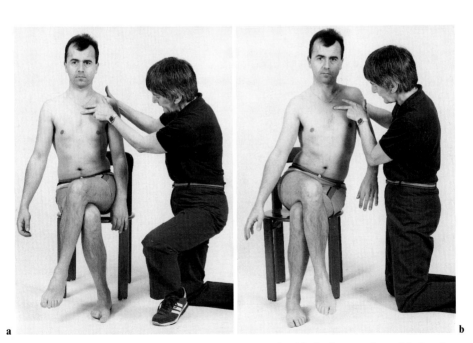

a   b

Fig. 6.37 a, b. Selective lateral flexion of the lower trunk with the foot on the weight-bearing side flat on the floor (left hemiplegia). **a** Weight over the sound side. **b** Weight over the hemiplegic side

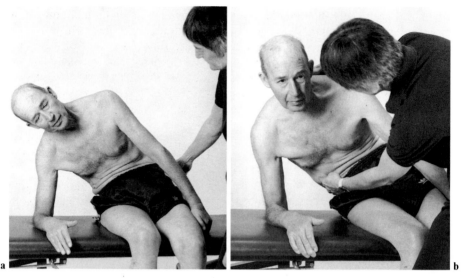

Fig. 6.38 a, b. Active side flexion of the trunk against gravity when returning to an upright sitting position (left hemiplegia). **a** Incorrect starting position. **b** Adjusting the position of the head and trunk

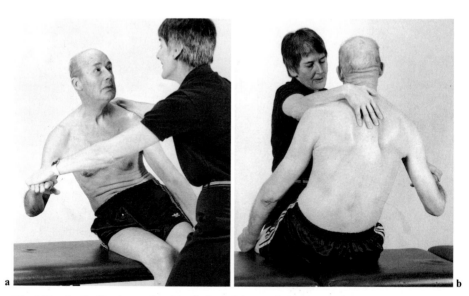

Fig. 6.39 a, b. Facilitating active side flexion of the trunk against gravity as the patient moves to and from an upright sitting position (left hemiplegia). **a** The therapist holds the sound hand lightly from above to keep it off the plinth. **b** Her forearm pushes downwards over the hemiplegic side to stimulate lateral flexion of the neck and trunk

which is placed round behind his shoulder. When leaning on their sound elbow most patients will shorten the underside of their trunk, and the hemiplegic side elongates (Fig. 6.38a). The muscle activity will be changed as a result when returning to the vertical. The therapist takes time to correct the starting position. She instructs the patient to lower his ribs on the underside towards the supporting surface, indicating the part with her hand (Fig. 6.38b). She also adjusts the position of the head towards the hemiplegic side. The patient is asked to sit up again, and the therapist pushes down on his hemiplegic shoulder with her forearm to stimulate lateral flexion of his neck and trunk. Her other hand holds his sound hand lightly from above and reminds him not to use it to assist the movement (Fig. 6.39a,b).

As the patient's trunk control improves, the therapist can interrupt the movement, either on the way down or the way up, and the muscle activity is increased as more prolonged holding is required.

6.7 Moving Forwards and Backwards

When adjusting his position on a plinth or bed, the patient learns to walk on his buttocks, either backwards or forwards as required. If the movement is not carefully taught, the patient will pull himself into position using his sound hand. The activity is, as a result, very one sided, and almost inevitably his hemi-

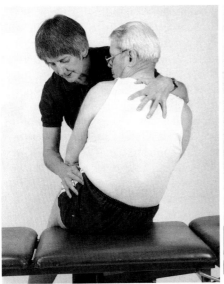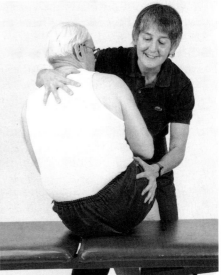

Fig. 6.40 a, b. Assisting the patient to move backwards and forwards in sitting (left hemiplegia). **a** With weight over the sound side, the hemiplegic hip is helped to move. **b** With weight taken well over to the hemiplegic side, the opposite hip is moved

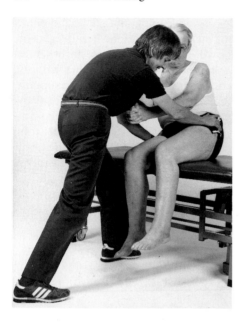

Fig. 6.41. Moving first one buttock and then the other in the required direction with less support (left hemiplegia)

plegic leg will extend strongly in the spastic pattern of extension. Instead he should clasp his hands together in the midline and move first one buttock and then the other in the desired direction.

The therapist facilitates the correct movement by standing in front of the patient and placing one hand beneath the buttock which is to be moved. Her other hand is behind his shoulder on the contralateral side to enable him to transfer his weight towards that side and to maintain his trunk in an upright position. She helps him to lift his buttock off the surface and to move it backwards or forwards (Fig. 6.40a). She changes her hands each time to the opposite side to assist the movement of the other buttock (Fig. 6.40b).

As the patient takes over the movement the therapist gives less support. Once he can maintain an upright position, she facilitates the activity with her hands, one on each side of his pelvis, assisting the rotation. The patient keeps his hands clasped in front of him throughout as he moves back and forth (Fig. 6.41).

Finally, he learns to walk backwards or forwards on his buttocks automatically whenever he is moving in sitting (Fig. 6.42a, b).

6.8 Conclusion

Certain activities in daily life can be used to improve abdominal muscle activity if performed more normally. As has been described in the previous chapter, the

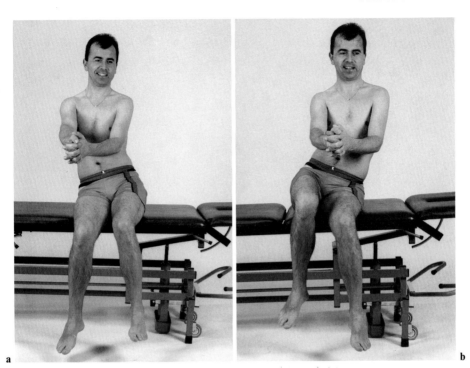

Fig. 6.42 a, b. Moving in sitting unaided by walking backwards or forwards on the buttocks (left hemiplegia)

patient can learn to come to sitting from lying without pulling himself upright with his sound hand, but by using his trunk muscles instead. When crossing one leg over the other as he may need to do when putting on his trousers or shoes, he learns to do so actively, instead of lifting the affected leg with the help of his sound hand. The movement is more selective if he keeps his trunk erect while flexing the leg to place it over the other one. If possible, the patient learns to put on his socks and shoes while holding his leg in the air with active flexion instead of crossing one over the other. Whether he is doing so with the hemiplegic hand assisting the activity or with the sound hand alone, it is important that the leg is between his arms and not being held in a position of abduction and outward rotation (Fig. 6.43 a, b). With the knee held in front of him the lumbar spine is flexed and the lower abdominals activated (Fig. 6.43 c, d). The foot of the other leg should remain flat on the floor. The therapist should observe the patient as he performs activities of daily living and see if she can teach him to do some in a more therapeutic way.

Learning to ride a bicycle can be a pleasant hobby and is also a most effective form of stimulating trunk activity and balance (Fig. 6.44). More disabled patients may only be able to manage a bicycle with balance wheels at the back (Fig. 6.45).

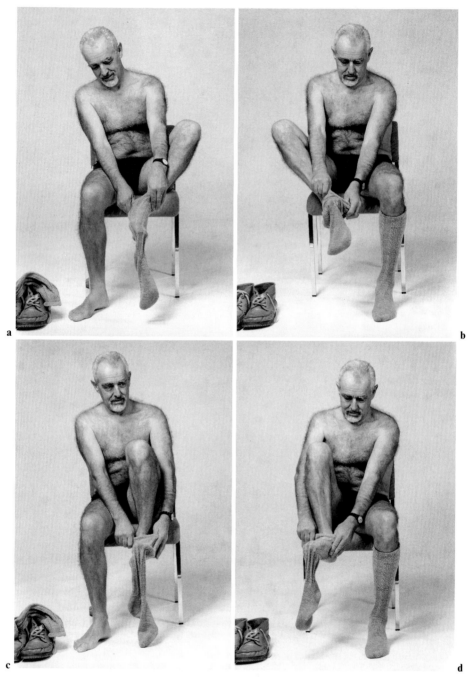

Fig. 6.43 a–d. Putting on shoes and socks with the leg held actively in the air (right hemiplegia). **a, b** With outward rotation and abduction of the hip, the lower abdominals are not activated. **c, d** With the knee between the arms the lumbar spine flexes and the lower abdominal muscles hold actively

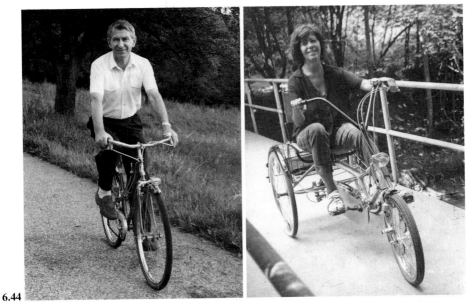

6.44

6.45

Fig. 6.44. Learning to ride a bicycle is enjoyable and stimulates trunk activity as well (right hemiplegia), (Compare with Figs. 3.23 a and 3.39 b)

Fig. 6.45. A more disabled patient may need a tricycle with a seat instead of a saddle at first in order to enjoy the countryside (right hemiplegia). (Compare with Figs. 3.29 a and 3.35 a)

7 Standing Up from Sitting

Patients have difficulty in standing up from sitting in a normal way as the movement requires selective activity of the trunk and the legs simultaneously. Normally when we stand up, the extended trunk is brought forwards so far that our head is over our feet or even further. As the trunk moves forwards, the extensor muscles of the hips and knees are active, and then as our seat leaves the supporting surface the knees move forward over our feet at first. The ankles are therefore required to dorsiflex further, even though there is increased activity in the hip and knee extensors (Fig. 7.1). Both hips maintain the same degree of rotation and abduction so that the knees move neither towards nor away from one another (Fig. 7.2). The arms swing slightly forward with the momentum caused by the trunk moving forwards; only when we stand up from a low stool

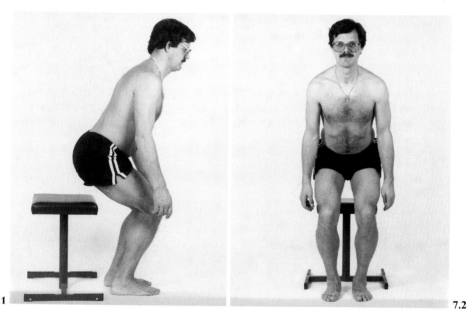

7.1   7.2

Fig. 7.1. Standing up from sitting requires selective extensor activity in the trunk and legs (normal model)

Fig. 7.2. When standing up from sitting the knees move neither towards nor away from one another, and the arms swing slightly forward with momentum (normal model)

do we use our extended arms actively in order to bring more weight forwards (Fig. 7.3). Standing up from sitting is a very important activity for the patient because if he does so in an abnormal way, he will be reinforcing a mass movement synergy, and through constant repetition extensor spasticity in his leg will be increased as a result. If he stands up incorrectly, his first steps will also be abnormal. When practised correctly the activity is most useful for retraining selective movement of the legs and the trunk, which in turn will improve the patient's walking pattern.

The three most common difficulties for the patient are:

1. He cannot extend this trunk when his hips are flexed, nor flex his hips sufficiently while extensor activity is required (Fig. 7.4). He is therefore not able to bring his weight far enough forward over his feet.

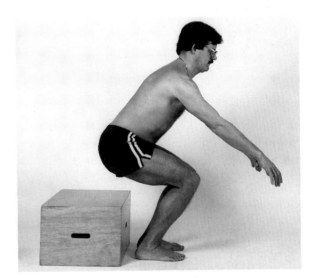

Fig. 7.3. The arms extend actively only if the seat is very low (normal model)

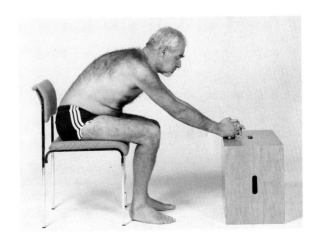

Fig. 7.4. The patient has difficulty in extending his trunk when his hips are flexed and in flexing his hips when extensor activity is required (right hemiplegia)

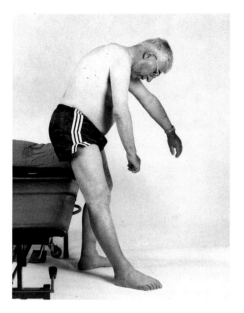

Fig. 7.5. A patient stands up incorrectly using the total mass pattern of extension of his leg, which prevents his weight from being brought far enough forwards (right hemiplegia)

2. The hemiplegic hip adducts because extensor activity is needed, and it is not possible for the patient without the adduction component of the extensor synergy. The heel of the hemiplegic limb may leave the floor, as plantar flexion occurs together with the extension at the knee.
3. Because the patient has been unable to bring his weight far enough forward, and because his hip extensors and plantar flexors are acting simultaneously in the total mass synergy, he pushes backwards in his effort to stand up, his knee moving backwards instead of forwards (Fig. 7.5).

During the activities performed to overcome these problems and in order to regain selective activity of the muscle groups involved, the therapist must facilitate the normal movement pattern and prevent these abnormal movement components from occurring.

7.1 Therapeutic and Functional Activities

7.1.1 Bringing the Extended Trunk Forwards

The therapist places her foot on a stool directly in front of the patient. She rests the patient's extended arms on her thigh, his elbows or upper arms being supported in such a way that the shoulder is kept aligned. The therapist uses one hand to press the spine into extension. The other hand gives counter-pressure on the patient's chest or it can support his shoulder if necessary. By abducting

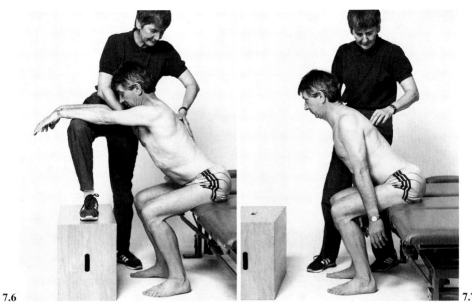

7.6   7.7

Fig. 7.6. Regaining extension of the trunk with the arms supported. The patient's hands should not be clasped together as the resultant flexion hampers extension of the thoracic spine (right hemiplegia)

Fig. 7.7. Maintaining active extension of the spine as the trunk is brought forwards (right hemiplegia)

her leg the therapist enables the patient to move his trunk further forward while still maintaining extension of the spine (Fig. 7.6).

After the preparatory extension with supported arms, the patient leaves his arms at his sides and moves his trunk forwards actively, the therapist helping him, as required, to maintain the extension (Fig. 7.7). She may need to use her leg to help him to maintain his knee over his foot.

Some patients may find the extension of the spine impossible at first, even without leaning forwards. To give more assistance the therapist places one of her knees against the patient's spine at the level of the kyphosis and uses her hands to help him to bring his shoulders back. She asks him to bring the appropriate part of his back away from her knee, and so gives him a clear point of reference. Using the same facilitation she then encourages the patient to lean forwards and return to the upright position repeatedly, going further forwards each time (Fig. 7.8). The patient should only go as far forwards as he can without losing the extension of his spine.

Some patients, particularly those whose hip adducts as they bring their trunk forward (Fig. 7.9) may find it easier to learn the movement if they first bend forward completely and then extend their spine without extending their hips.

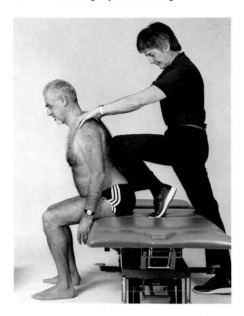

Fig. 7.8. Facilitating trunk extension as the patient leans forwards (right hemiplegia)

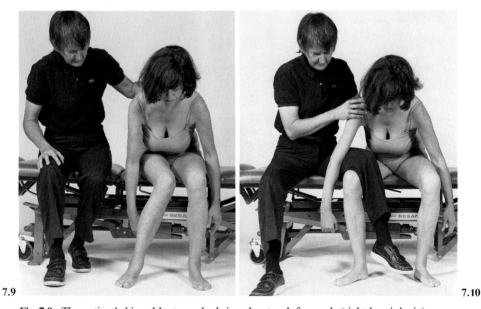

7.9

7.10

Fig. 7.9. The patient's hip adducts as she brings her trunk forwards (right hemiplegia)

Fig. 7.10. Preventing adduction of the hip when the patient brings her trunk forwards (right hemiplegia)

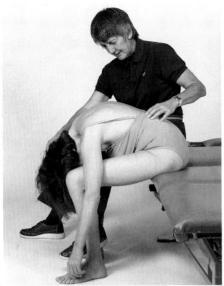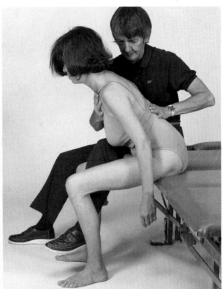

Fig. 7.11 a, b. Facilitating selective extension of the trunk and hemiplegic leg (right hemiplegia). **a** The patient relaxes, bent completely forwards with her arms hanging loosely. **b** The therapist holds the hemiplegic leg in abduction and assists trunk extension

The therapist sits beside the patient on his affected side. She places her leg over his thigh and keeps the hip abducted and his knee over his foot. The pressure of her leg also prevents the patient's heel from pushing up off the floor as he leans forward (Fig. 7.10).

The patient bends forward with his nose in the middle of the space between his legs and his arms hanging loosely until his hands touch his feet. He should be encouraged to let his head hang forward with his neck relaxed as well (Fig. 7.11a). When he has bent forward and returned to a sitting position several times the therapist will notice that his leg is no longer pulling into adduction and can reduce the amount of support she needs to give with her leg. The patient is also asked to let his leg remain where it is without pulling and to leave his foot consciously flat on the floor without it pushing.

Leaving her leg over his, the therapist instructs the patient to straighten his back without coming up to a sitting position. With one of her hands placed against his sternum she helps him to extend his thoracic spine. Her other hand applies counter-pressure over the lumbar spine and prevents his body from moving backwards (Fig. 7.11b). The patient should keep his head in line with his spine and not overextend his neck as he extends his back.

Keeping his back straight in the corrected position he returns to an upright position and then brings his extended trunk forwards, the axis of the movement being his hip joints. No flexion should occur at any level of his spine.

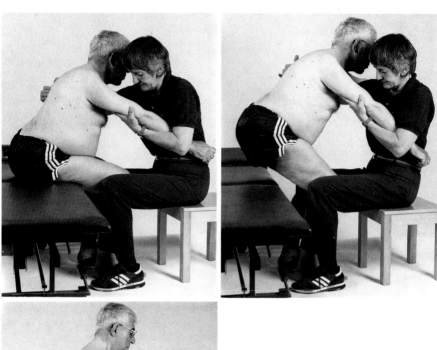

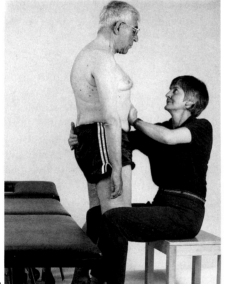

Fig. 7.12 a–c. Facilitating the activity of standing up from sitting (right hemiplegia). **a** The therapist holds the patient's hemiplegic knee between hers and supports his affected arm. **b** She draws his knee forward over his foot and assists trunk extension. **c** She adjusts the position of his pelvis

7.1.2 Standing Up from Sitting

7.1.2.1 Supported by the Therapist

If the activity is still very difficult for the patient, the therapist may need to give a considerable amount of help to ensure a normal movement pattern. She sits in front of the patient and holds his hemiplegic knee between her knees, so that

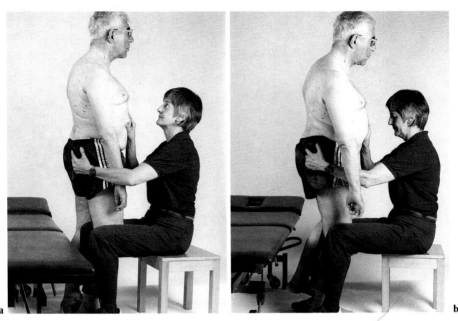

a   b

Fig. 7.13 a, b. Transferring weight over the hemiplegic leg (right hemiplegia). **a** With her knees the therapist guides the patient's weight towards the hemiplegic side. **b** The patient lifts his foot off the floor

she can control the forward movement of the knee over the foot as well as the necessary abduction of the hip. She tells the patient not to attempt to stand up, but merely to lean forward towards her. She places his hemiplegic hand under her arm on that side and holds his upper arm gently in oder to protect his shoulder. With her other hand the therapist helps the patient to extend his thoracic spine by indicating the kyphotic area, usually at about T8–T10 (Fig. 7.12 a). After he has extended his spine, the therapist then asks the patient to lift his buttocks from the supporting surface without pushing back against her hand. She uses her knees to draw his knee forwards, at the same time preventing his heel from leaving the floor (Fig. 7.12 b). Her hand on his thoracic spine also helps to facilitate the forward movement required. As the patient stands up the therapist releases his hemiplegic arm and helps him to extend his hips, one of her hands assisting the hip extensors, the other the action of the lower abdominals to tilt his pelvis up at the front (Fig. 7.12 c). From her position in front of the patient, the therapist can then assist him wherever necessary as she has both her hands free (Fig. 7.13 a). With her knees she can help him to transfer his weight over his hemiplegic leg without allowing the knee to push back into hyperextension even when he lifts his sound foot from the floor (Fig. 7.13 b).

When the therapist helps the patient to sit down again, she uses much the same facilitation as she did to enable him to stand up. She holds his hemiplegic arm against her body and enables him to lower his seat slowly to the plinth by

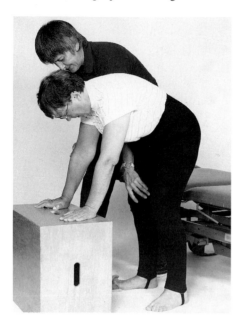

Fig. 7.14. Standing up with the hands supported on a stool. The therapist holds the hemiplegic elbow in extension and assists the movement of the knee (right hemiplegia)

keeping his weight well forward with her other hand on his thoracic spine. The movement of the trunk proximally against the spastic arm inhibits its flexor hypertonicity and prepares the arm for more active participation.

7.1.2.2 Hands Supported on a Stool

The therapist helps the patient to place both his hands flat on a stool directly in front of him. If necessary, she holds his elbow in extension, applying some downward pressure to ensure that his hand remains in position as he lifts his seat off the supporting surface and brings his weight forwards over his arms (Fig. 7.14). With her other hand the therapist guides the patient's knee over his foot, so that the active extension of the leg takes place without the hip adducting. A rolled bandage under the patient's toes inhibits their flexion.

Maintaining his knees in a slightly flexed position the patient extends his spine and then rounds his back (Fig. 7.15 a, b). The angle of flexion at the knee remains constant as he flexes and extends his trunk.

With his back extended, the patient moves his pelvis selectively from one side to the other, using the side flexors of his lumbar spine to do so. The therapist stabilises the patient's thorax between her body and her upper arm, using her hands to facilitate the lateral movement of the pelvis in isolation (Fig. 7.16 a, b).

The patient places his hands flat on the floor in front of him and then raises his buttocks off the plinth. The therapist assists in maintaining elbow extension and preventing adduction of the hip (Fig. 7.17 a, b).

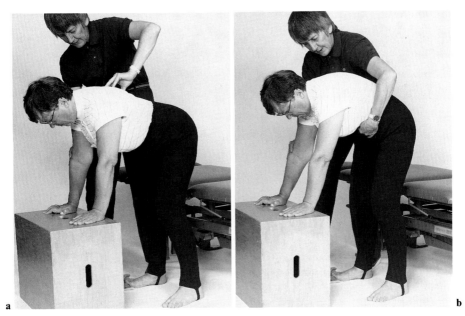

Fig. 7.15 a, b. Moving the trunk actively with weight taken through both arms (right hemiplegia). **a** Extending the spine. **b** Flexing the spine without altering the position of the knees

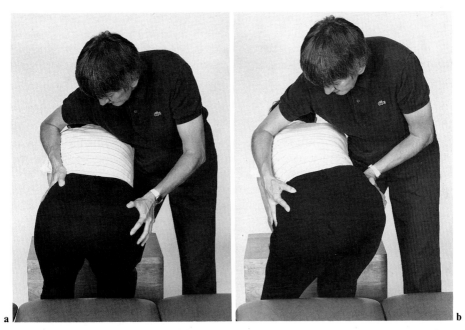

Fig. 7.16 a, b. Selective lateral flexion of the trunk with weight taken through both arms (right hemiplegia). **a** The therapist holds the hemiplegic arm in extension with her leg and helps the patient to stabilise her thorax. **b** Her hands facilitate the lateral movement of the pelvis

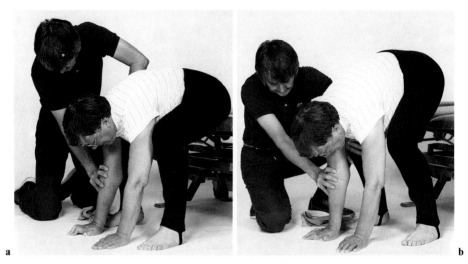

a   b

Fig. 7.17 a, b. Retraining selective extensor activity of the hemiplegic leg with both hands flat on the floor (right hemiplegia). **a** Adjusting the starting position. **b** The patient lifts her seat off the plinth

If the activity is difficult for the patient at first, the height of a stool in front of him can be gradually reduced until he can perform the movement with his hands on the floor. It is usually easier for him to start by lowering his seat to the plinth when the height of the stool is reduced than to raise his buttocks from sitting. After lowering his seat, the activity needed to extend his legs concentrically becomes possible (Fig. 7.18 a, b).

7.1.2.3 Weight Bearing on the Hemiplegic Leg Alone

The patient crosses his sound leg over the hemiplegic leg and lifts his seat from the plinth. The therapist places one arm across his back and facilitates the movement with her hand over his trochanter. Her shoulder behind him prevents his trunk from pushing backwards (Fig. 7.19 a). A stool or chair placed in front of the patient gives him the confidence to lean far enough forwards as he knows he can use his sound hand to regain his balance if necessary.

Once the patient can bear weight on his leg in this position, the therapist asks him to extend his back (Fig. 7.19 b). He can also practise flexing and extending the supporting knee. The activity is useful in that it ensures selective extension in the weight-bearing hemiplegic leg. The sound leg crossed over the other prevents the heel from leaving the floor and ensures dorsal flexion at the ankle, despite the active extension at the knee and hip. A rolled bandage under the patient's toes holds them in dorsal extension, thus preventing them from flexing in the mass pattern of extension. The trunk side flexors are activated selectively in order to maintain balance on such a narrow base.

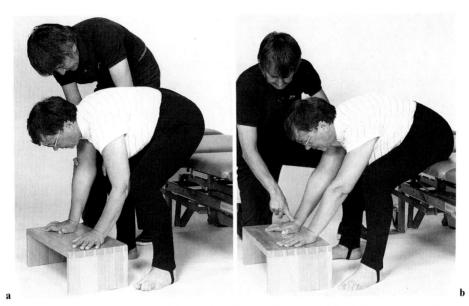

Fig. 7.18 a, b. Learning to extend the hemiplegic leg selectively with both hands supported on a low stool (right hemiplegia). **a** The therapist helps to maintain elbow extension and corrects the position of the hemiplegic knee. **b** The patient lowers her seat to the plinth

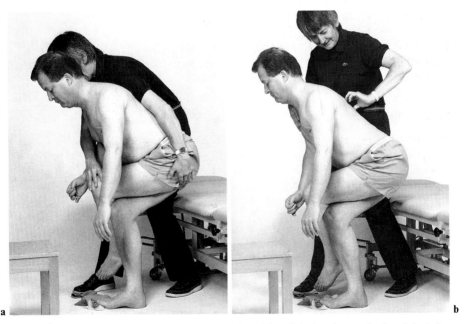

Fig. 7.19 a, b. Facilitating selective extensor activity with weight bearing on the hemiplegic leg alone (right hemiplegia). **a** With the sound leg crossed over the other one, the patient is helped to lift his seat off the plinth. **b** He maintains his balance while extending his trunk

7.1.3 Alternating Between Selective Extensor and Flexor Activity of the Trunk and Hips

Preparation for the following sequence of activities can be started as soon as the patient starts sitting out of bed, regardless of the degree of his disability. As his ability improves, the sequence can be gradually progressed, and the selective activity which the patient regains as a result will help him to stand up and walk more normally.

The patient supports his arms on a table placed in front of him and is frequently unable to extend his spine sufficiently (Fig. 7.20).

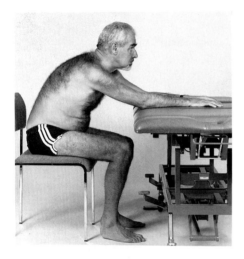

Fig. 7.20. Difficulty in extending the trunk even when the arms are supported on a table (right hemiplegia)

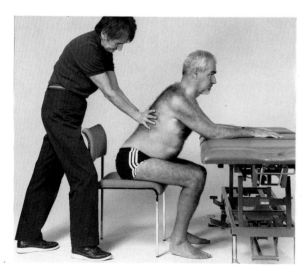

Fig. 7.21. Regaining passive extension of the spine (right hemiplegia)

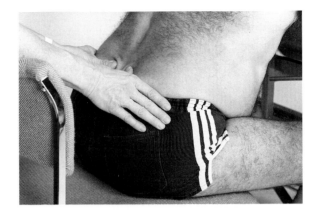

Fig. 7.22. Helping the patient to extend his lower lumbar spine (right hemiplegia)

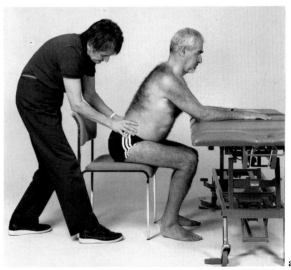

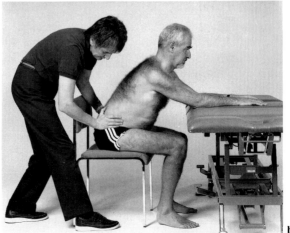

Fig. 7.23 a, b. Extending and flexing the lumbar spine selectively (right hemiplegia)

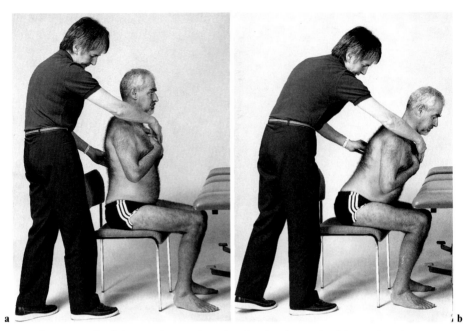

a   b

Fig. 7.24 a, b. Maintaining trunk extension when leaning forwards (right hemiplegia)

The therapist presses down on his back gently but firmly and moves his spine passively into extension (Fig. 7.21).

Once he can extend his thoracic spine, the therapist helps the patient to extend his spine at the lumbosacral junction. She presses her thumbs against the kyphotic area which can almost always be observed over the level of the fifth lumbar vertebrae (Fig. 7.22). The patient takes over the movement actively and then flexes and extends the lumbar spine alternately, while stabilising his thoracic spine. The movement becomes increasingly selective and the pelvis more mobile (Fig. 7.23 a, b).

The patient places his hands on his chest, the sound hand over the hemiplegic one. He moves his extended trunk forwards from the hips, without allowing any flexion to occur in the spine (Fig. 7.24a, b). His hands can also be left at his sides as he moves. The therapist helps him to stabilise his trunk in the extended position by placing one hand over his hands on his sternum and her other assisting the extension of the thoracic spine. The patient is asked to keep his head in line with his trunk as he will usually extend his neck over-actively in an attempt to extend his trunk. Once he can perform the movement backwards and forwards without the therapist's hand on his sternum, she can use her hand to prevent the hip from adducting and help the patient to keep his knee over his foot (Fig. 7.25). When the patient can move his extended trunk freely and easily, the table or plinth in front of him is no longer necessary. A stool in front of him is still useful, however, to give him the confidence to lean far enough forward, as he will need to do when he lifts his seat off the plinth.

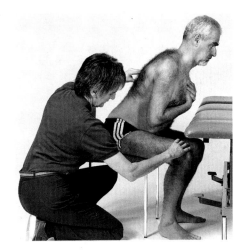

Fig. 7.25. Preventing adduction of the hemiplegic hip when the extended trunk moves forwards (right hemiplegia)

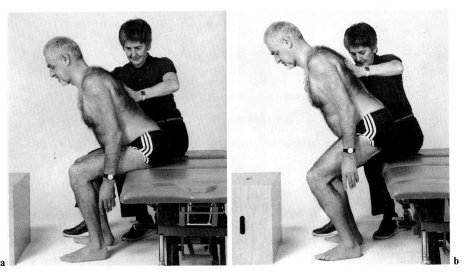

Fig. 7.26 a, b. Facilitating trunk extension with weight bearing on both legs (right hemiplegia). **a** The therapist places one hand on the patient's sternum, the other over his thoracic spine. **b** The patient lifts his seat off the plinth

The patient brings his extended trunk forward until his head is well over his feet, his arms remaining at his sides. The therapist once again helps to stabilise his trunk with one of her hands on his sternum, the other on the thoracic spine (Fig. 7.26 a).

The patient lifts his seat off the plinth, but still keeps his trunk extended, only the hips flexing to bring the trunk forwards (Fig. 7.26 b).

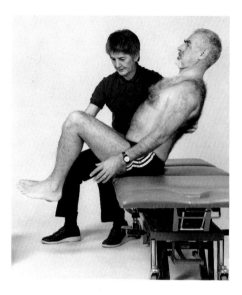

Fig. 7.27. Rocking backwards with both feet leaving the floor, and the hips and knees held at right angles (right hemiplegia).

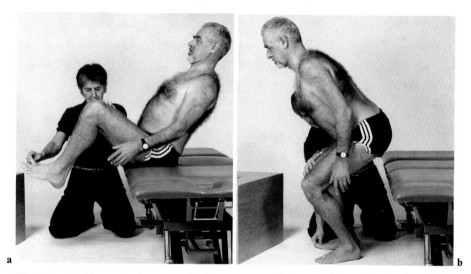

a   b

Fig. 7.28 a, b. Alternating between selective extensor and flexor activity of the trunk and hips. The therapist corrects the positions of the hemiplegic knee and foot (right hemiplegia). **a** Flexor activity. **b** Extensor activity

The patient lowers his seat to the plinth again and leans back, lifting his legs actively as he does so. He holds his hips, knees and feet all at right angles. At first the therapist will need to assist the hemiplegic leg in order to achieve the required angle at the knee and hip. As the patient rocks backwards she also uses one hand to assist the extension of the thoracic spine. The patient's head remains in line with his trunk (Fig. 7.27).

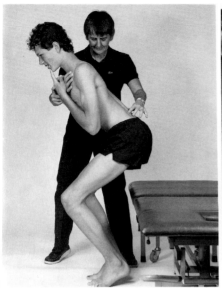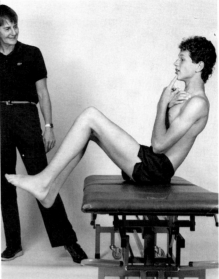

a   b

Fig. 7.29 a, b. Training active plantar flexion of the foot with weight bearing (right hemiplegia). **a** The patient keeps his knees over his feet as his seat leaves the plinth. **b** He tries to maintain trunk extension when his feet leave the floor

The patient repeats the movement sequence, rocking first forwards and lifting his seat off the plinth and then backwards again, with his legs flexing. The therapist will often need to support the patient's hemiplegic foot in dorsal flexion as it returns to the floor and also when the legs are flexed actively (Fig. 7.28 a, b).

Once the activity has been mastered, variations, each emphasising another aspect of selective activity, can be added and the degree of difficulty increased. For advanced patients the activities can be usefully included in the home programme.

7.1.3.1 Incorporating Active Plantar Flexion of the Foot

The patient rocks forwards and then backwards in the same way as before, but as he lifts his seat off the plinth he only takes his weight on the balls of his feet and his toes, using active plantar flexion of his ankles. His knees must remain over his feet. If the patient holds his hands on his chest and places the tip of the index finger of his sound hand on the front of his chin, he automatically keeps his head in the correct position (Fig. 7.29 a, b). The patient must attempt to prevent his lumbar spine from flexing at all during the backwards movement of his trunk. The activity trains active plantar flexion of the ankle together with selective extension of the knee in the weight-bearing phase. When the feet are lifted from the floor and the weight is transferred backwards, selective flexion of the legs is emphasised and selective extension of the trunk is maintained, despite the active hip flexion and strong lower abdominal muscle activity.

7.1.3.2 Legs Crossed

The patient crosses one leg in front of the other during the non-weight-bearing phase of the activity and brings his weight forward, with his feet remaining side by side in the new position. As he leans backwards again, he crosses the other leg in front. Weight bearing with crossed legs emphasises selective hip extension in that the hips must actively extend in outward rotation and without adducting (Fig. 7.30a, b). It also demands considerable activity from the trunk side flexors to maintain balance.

7.1.3.3 Performing an Additional Task

To allow the movement to become more automatic and effortless, the patient can continue the forward and backward movement, while at the same time performing another task, e. g. putting on his shirt (Fig. 7.31a, b) or reading a book.

7.1.4 Standing Up from a High Plinth or Bed

Activities in which the patient is helped to come to a standing position from a high plinth or bed can improve both selective extension in his leg as well as selective trunk control. The patient stands on one leg and lifts the contra-lateral hip up onto the plinth. The activity is also useful when lifting a patient back on to a bed or plinth if its height is not adjustable.

7.1.4.1 Transferring the Patient onto a High Bed

When the patient is still confined to a wheelchair and is unable to take sufficient weight on his hemiplegic leg, the therapist or nurse will need to give him full support in order to transfer him to a bed or plinth that cannot be lowered.

She brings the patient to stand leaning with his back against the bed. With one of her thighs in front of his hemiplegic knee and the other behind it, she draws the patient towards her, supporting his trunk with both her arms and stabilising his leg with her thighs (Fig. 7.32a).

The patient lifts his sound leg off the floor and the therapist places one of her hands beneath his thigh and lifts his buttock on that side on to the bed (Fig. 7.32b).

The patient's weight is supported on the bed as the therapist changes the position of her hands. One arm is placed around behind his sound shoulder to enable him to transfer his weight over to the unaffected side. With her other hand the therapist lifts the patient's hemiplegic leg and moves his buttock back onto the bed (Fig. 7.32c).

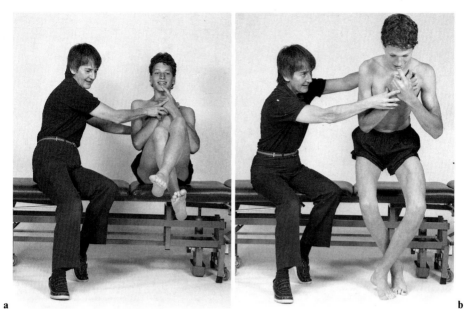

Fig. 7.30 a, b. Alternating between selective extensor and flexor activity of the trunk and hips with one leg crossing in front of the other (right hemiplegia) in **a** flexion and **b** extension

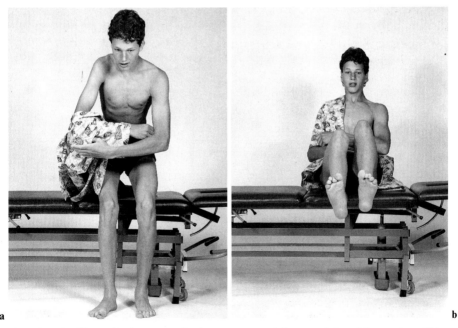

Fig. 7.31 a, b. Alternating between selective extensor and flexor activity of the trunk and hips while putting on a shirt (right hemiplegia)

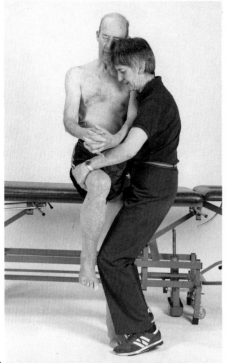

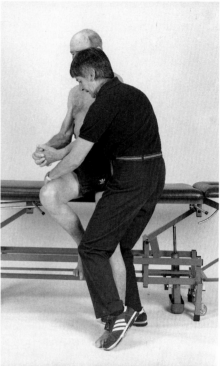

a

b

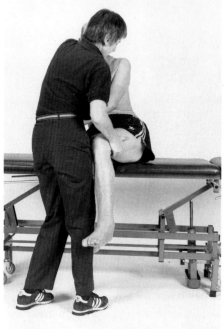

Fig. 7.32 a–c. Helping a wheel-chair patient on to a high plinth (left hemiplegia).
a The therapist holds the patient's hemiplegic knee between her thighs. **b** The sound buttock is lifted on to the plinth.
c The affected buttock is brought up on to the plinth

c

7.1.5 Standing Up and Returning to Sitting from a High Plinth or Bed

7.1.5.1 Weight Taken on the Hemiplegic Leg

When the patient is sitting on the plinth, the therapist kneels beside him and guides his hemiplegic foot slowly to the floor. The patient keeps his trunk erect and holds the weight of his hemiplegic leg actively, allowing the flexor muscle groups to play out gradually, without the leg pushing into extension. By holding his toes in full dorsal extension, the therapist helps to prevent the total extensor synergy from occurring, and the foot is placed flat on the floor (Fig. 7.33).

The therapist stands beside the patient and uses one of her hands to assist hip extension on the hemiplegic side, using the support described in Chap. 8. Her other arm is placed behind the patient with her hand over his waist as she helps him to stand up on his hemiplegic leg and lower his other foot slowly to the floor (Fig. 7.34a).

To return to sitting on the plinth the patient flexes his sound leg, taking care that his hemiplegic knee does not snap back into a hyper-extended position as he places his buttock on to the supporting surface behind him. The therapist assists the correct movement by keeping the patient's hemiplegic hip well forward, with his knee over his foot (Fig. 7.34b). The activity is repeated, back and forth, and also with the sound leg remaining in the air, not quite reaching the floor.

When the patient is able to perform the activity confidently and correctly, the therapist kneels in front of him as he comes off the plinth and returns to a

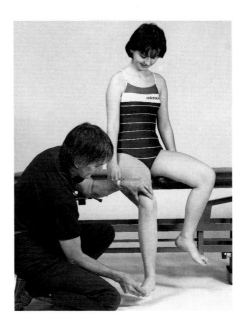

Fig. 7.33. Before standing up from a high plinth, the hemiplegic foot is placed flat on the floor (right hemiplegia)

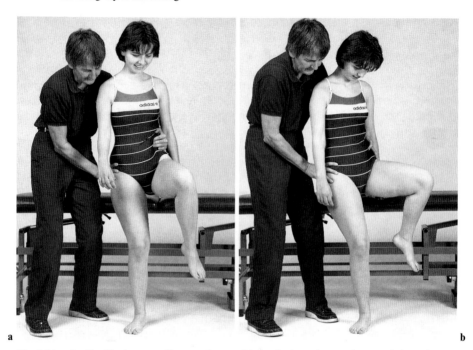

a   b

Fig. 7.34 a, b. Facilitating standing up from a high plinth and returning to sitting with the weight taken on the hemiplegic leg (right hemiplegia)

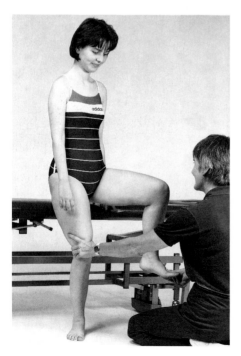

Fig. 7.35. Taking all the weight on the hemiplegic leg when standing up from a high plinth and returning to sitting (right hemiplegia)

sitting position again. She hold the toes of the sound foot lightly and indicates the direction of the movement back and forth. The patients comes to a standing position on his hemiplegic leg and, without placing the sound foot on the floor, is asked to return to sitting and then stand up again. With her other hand the therapist assists the patient's knee on the hemiplegic side, preventing it from rolling inwards as it will do if the hemiplegic hip adducts and inwardly rotates with extension (Fig. 7.35). The activity improves selective extension of the leg for the stance phase of walking.

7.1.5.2 Weight Taken on the Sound Leg

From a sitting position on the plinth, the patient brings his sound foot to the floor. At first the therapist will need to sit on a stool in front of him as she helps him to bring his hemiplegic foot down in a controlled way. Her leg, supporting the lateral side of his sound leg, will enable the patient to transfer his weight sufficiently over that side as it provides stability and a point of reference for the required amount of weight shift sideways. The therapist guides the patient as he comes to standing and returns to a sitting position again (Fig. 7.36). The patient's trunk should remain upright throughout the activity.

When the patient has learned the correct movement and feels confident, the therapist kneels at his feet and can give far less support. With one hand she holds the patient's hemiplegic foot, with the toes in dorsal extension, and helps

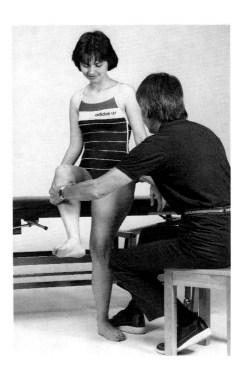

Fig. 7.36. Facilitating the movement of standing up and returning to sitting with weight taken on the sound leg (right hemiplegia)

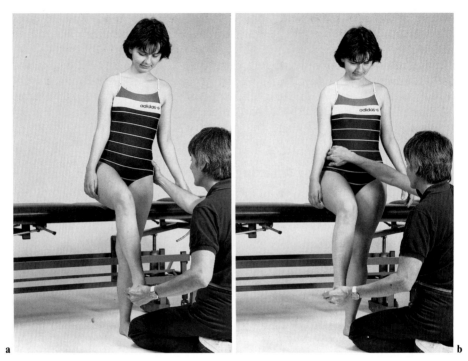

a   b

Fig. 7.37 a, b. Coming to standing from a high plinth with the weight on the sound leg (right hemiplegia). **a** The therapist holds the patient's hemiplegic foot in dorsiflexion. **b** She uses her hand to prevent elevation of the side of the pelvis as the foot is lowered to the floor

to prevent supination as he moves his leg (Fig. 7.37 a, b). Her other hand helps the patient to avoid hitching up the side of his pelvis when he flexes his hemi-plegic leg to move it back and forth.

The activity improves selective control of the trunk and the hemiplegic leg for the swing phase of walking.

7.2 Conclusion

Activities preparing the patient to stand up from sitting correctly are most use-ful for retraining selective control of the trunk and selective extension of the hemiplegic leg. When we lean forwards in sitting, our legs immediately func-tion as a support for the trunk, and the hip and knee extensors are activated. When we lift our seat from the supporting surface, the leg extensors are re-quired to act strongly to prevent flexion. Repeating the activities described in the chapter will build up tone and strengthen the patient's hip and knee exten-sors. Because of the position of the legs, with the knee flexed and the foot in dorsiflexion, the activity will be selective and the danger of increasing extensor spasticity in a total pattern is avoided. Patients at all stages of their rehabilitation will benefit from the activities. Even those who can already walk unaided will improve the quality of their gait. Patients who are still in a wheelchair will need adequate support from the therapist and careful progression of the activities.

8 Activities in Standing

The ability to stand confidently and erect requires considerable adjustment from the postural muscles of the trunk which act to control the long mobile lever of the vertebral column or the series of small levers which constitute it. Standing erect also requires adequate muscle activity in the lower limbs to bear the weight of the body above. Despite the stabilising activity of the muscles around the hips, the pelvis must remain freely movable. For balance and the performance of functional activities in a standing position, the trunk cannot be fixed in a certain posture to compensate for inadequate musculature in the legs. The head, likewise, must remain freely movable. Mobile standing is a pre-requisite for normal walking.

Activities in standing are very important in the treatment programme and have the advantage of training simultaneously correct weight bearing on the hemiplegic leg. The more the patient stands with the assistance of the therapist, the less afraid he will be of the unaccustomed height. During the early stages following the onset of hemiplegia he may have spent considerable time lying in bed or sitting in a wheelchair fully supported. When he first stands up the floor may therefore seem to be a very long way away!

Disturbed sensory feedback will cause the patient to feel unsure when standing because the only certain contact he has with his surroundings is the sole of his sound foot on the floor. The control necessary for positioning the other parts of his body is dependent upon information provided by his own sensory system from within, and such information is often confusing and inaccurate. The patient will need to become accustomed to the new height again and relearn the feeling of the normal standing posture.

8.1 Important Considerations Before Standing Activities Are Begun

Before the patient is expected to stand, careful preparation of the necessary muscle activity is required, both in lying and in sitting positions, particularly selective extension of the hip and knee. If the patient has insufficient extensor tonus and active control, he will be forced to use the total pattern of extension, including plantar flexion of the foot or a compensatory mechanism with which he locks his knee into hyperextension by leaning his trunk forwards and flexing his hip. Activities preparing the patient for standing have been described in the previous chapters and by Davies (1985).

Because of the many joints involved, the possibilities for compensatory or alternative movements are manifold. The therapist needs to observe very critically to ensure that the various parts of the body are correctly positioned. The slightest deviation in posture can make a difference to the muscle activity.

The therapist should assist the patient in such a way that he does not need to support himself with his sound arm. The activity in the arm will otherwise take over the work of the trunk, and correct and relevant control will not be achieved.

The more the patient's tactile-kinaesthetic perception is disturbed, the more information he will need from his surroundings. Actual solid objects, such as a table placed in front of him, will help him to orientate the position of his body in space. Instructions such as "keep your thigh against the table" or "move your hip until it touches the table" are far easier for him to follow than "keep your hip forwards" or "shift your weight to the left".

The activities should be practised with the patient barefooted, so that the movements of the foot and toes can be observed and included in the treatment. Full extensibility of the Achilles tendon and the flexors of the toes can be

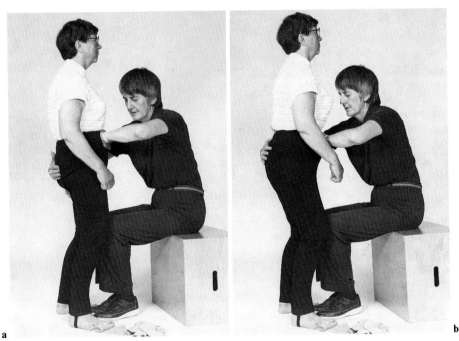

a   b

Fig. 8.1 a, b. Facilitating selective movement of the pelvis forwards and backwards (right hemiplegia). **a** The therapist places one hand over the patient's hip extensors and the other over her lower abdominal muscles. **b** Her knees keep the patient's hips in abduction and outward rotation

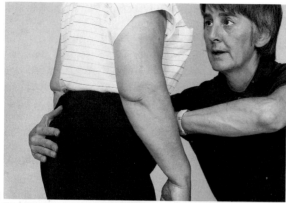

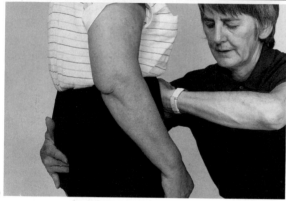

Fig. 8.2 a, b. Stabilising the thoracic spine while the lumbar spine is **a** extending and **b** flexing (right hemiplegia)

maintained and spasticity inhibited. The slightest contracture in the Achilles tendon will affect walking considerably as any shortening will prevent the patient from bringing his weight forward over his foot during the stance phase. As a result he will have to use compensatory postures of his head, trunk, knee and hip. A rolled bandage placed underneath the patient's toes during weight-bearing activities will inhibit distal spasticity and maintain the length of the Achilles tendon and the toe flexors.

8.2 Activities to Train Selective Trunk and Leg Movement

8.2.1 Tilting the Pelvis Forwards and Backwards

The patient stands with his weight on both legs and his knees slightly flexed (approximately 20°). The therapist sits on a stool in front of him and uses her knees to keep his legs abducted and outwardly rotated, so that his knees are pointing over his feet. She places one hand over his buttocks and the other over his lower abdominal muscles to facilitate the isolated movement of his pelvis

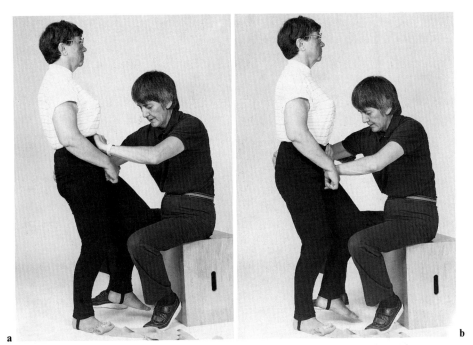

Fig. 8.3 a, b. Moving the pelvis rhythmically back and forth with the sound foot lifted off the floor (right hemiplegia)

forwards and backwards (Fig. 8.1 a, b). The patient keeps his knees in the same position, despite the movement of his pelvis. He also tries to stabilise the thoracic spine while the lumbar spine is flexing and extending (Fig. 8.2 a, b).

When the pelvis is moving freely and rhythmically back and forth the patient transfers his weight over the hemiplegic leg, without interrupting the pelvic movement. The movement continues even when he lifts his sound foot off the floor (Fig. 8.3 a, b). The patient is asked to hold the sound knee completely still in front of him as he will otherwise swing it backwards and forwards, using it to tilt his pelvis, instead of doing so with the muscles of the affected side.

8.2.2 Weight Bearing on the Hemiplegic Leg with Abduction and Adduction of the Contra-lateral Hip

The patient flexes his knees slightly and moves his weight over to the hemiplegic side. The therapist sits on a stool in front and somewhat to that side of him. Her leg outside his hemiplegic leg indicates how far he must shift his weight, i. e. until the lateral border of his leg is firmly against her leg. The therapist corrects the patient's posture with her hands, one of which helps him to extend his affected hip and the other to tense his abdominal muscles (Fig. 8.4).

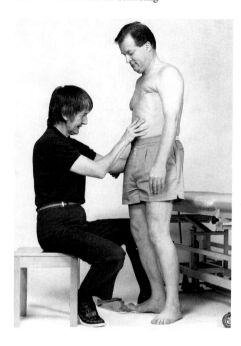

Fig. 8.4. Correcting the starting position for weight bearing on the hemiplegic leg with abduction and adduction of the contralateral hip (right hemiplegia)

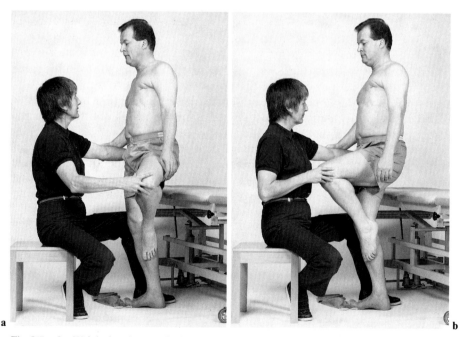

a   b

Fig. 8.5 a, b. Weight bearing on the hemiplegic leg with abduction and adduction of the contralateral hip. The sound foot is placed on the medial aspect of the hemiplegic knee (right hemiplegia). **a** Abduction with outward rotation. **b** Adduction with inward rotation

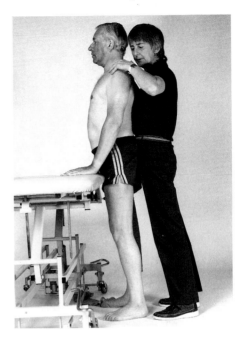

Fig. 8.6. Standing fully extended with the thighs against a plinth (right hemiplegia)

The patient then places his sound foot on the medial aspect of his hemiplegic knee, and without changing the position of his trunk, pelvis or weight-bearing leg he outwardly rotates his sound leg in abduction and then adducts it with inward rotation (Fig. 8.5 a, b).

8.2.3 Bending the Trunk Forwards and Bringing It to the Vertical Again

The patient stands with both his thighs against a plinth or table placed in front of him, its height such that it reaches approximately the level of his hips. The therapist stands behind him, pushing his seat forwards and straightening up his back and shoulders (Fig. 8.6). If he is unable to extend his knee adequately, or if he can only extend it with plantar flexion of his foot and toes, a splint should be used to hold his knee in extension. The simple splint is made of a hard material such as plaster of Paris, plastic or canvas with metal supports and should be bandaged firmly into place with a slightly elastic bandage (Fig. 8.7 a, b, c). The purpose of the splint is to hold the patient's knee in extension, without his having to make an effort to do so, either by pushing down with his foot or letting his hip move backwards. If is a useful adjuvant to treatment also for patients who have too little active movement or sensation in their hemiplegic leg. Those who have ankle clonus or even shortening of the Achilles tendon will benefit from weight bearing with the splint in situ and having their weight brought forwards with an increasing amount of dorsal flexion of the ankle.

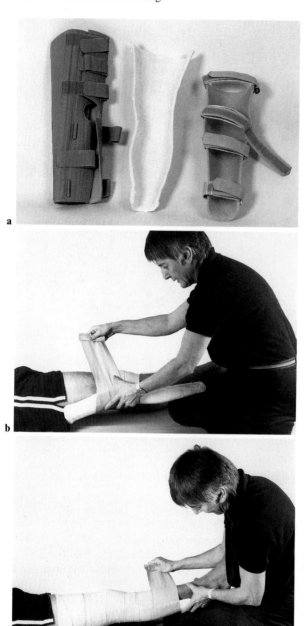

a

b

c

Fig. 8.7 a–c. Using a splint to hold the knee in extension. **a** Knee extension splints. **b** The therapist first bandages the knee firmly in the splint. **c** The bandage covers the whole splint (right hemiplegia)

The therapist reduces the amount of help she is giving and asks the patient to keep his thighs in contact with the plinth actively. Her other hand is placed over his sternum, assisting extension of his trunk (Fig. 8.8).

With his sound hand supported lightly on the plinth and his body upright,

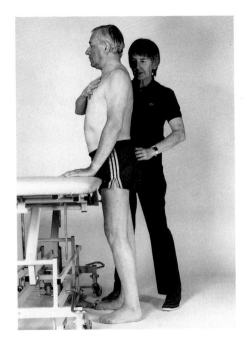

Fig. 8.8. Helping the patient to keep his hips forwards while extending his trunk (right hemiplegia)

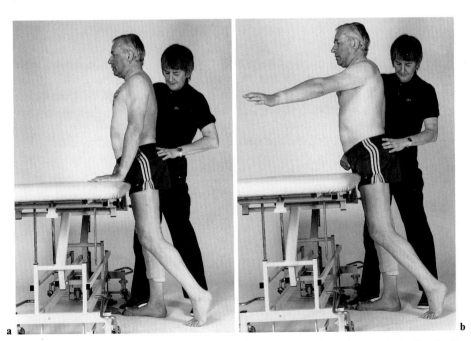

a

b

Fig. 8.9 a, b. Taking a step back with the sound leg and then lifting the supporting hand off the plinth (right hemiplegia)

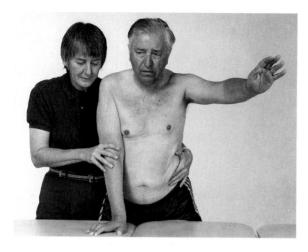

Fig. 8.10. Inhibiting spasticity in the hemiplegic arm (right hemiplegia)

the patient takes a step back with his sound foot, his thighs maintaining contact with the plinth (Fig. 8.9 a).

He lifts his sound arm up in front of him without changing the position of his trunk (Fig. 8.9 b).

Once he is able to repeat the sequence of movements without too much difficulty, the therapist can place his hemiplegic hand flat on the surface of the plinth and hold his arm in extension in order to inhibit flexor spasticity and encourage extensor activity (Fig. 8.10).

Standing at first with his feet parallel again, the patient clasps his hands together, and the therapist helps him to bring his elbows down to the plinth with his sound knee as straight as possible (Fig. 8.11 a). Still keeping his thighs against the plinth, the patient is asked to return to the upright position without pushing off with his elbow. His neck remains flexed until he is standing erect once more and should not push back into extension (Fig. 8.11 b).

Placing his sound foot behind him, the patient repeats the movement. The therapist ensures that the hemiplegic thigh does not lose contact with the plinth (Fig. 8.12 a, b).

8.2.4 Bending the Trunk Forwards and Returning to an Upright Position While Standing on a Sloping Surface

The patient stands on a wedge-shaped board with the plinth in front of him. A rolled bandage beneath his toes accentuates the effect of the sloping surface, increasing dorsal flexion of the ankle and toes (Fig. 8.13).

The therapist corrects the position of his trunk and asks him to move slightly away from the plinth and then towards it again, the only axis of movement being the ankle joints.

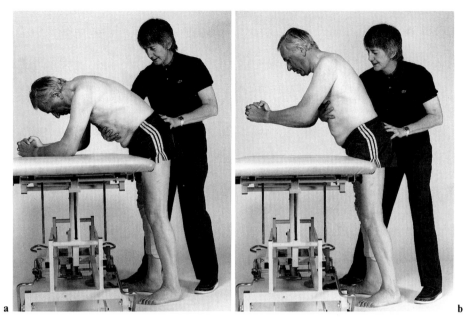

Fig. 8.11 a, b. Bringing both elbows down to the plinth and returning to an upright position (right hemiplegia). **a** With his hands clasped together the patient places his elbows on the plinth. **b** Standing up again without pushing off with his hands

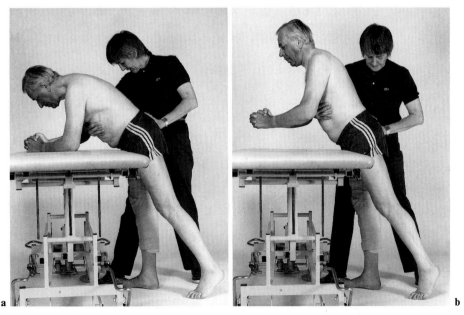

Fig. 8.12 a, b. Bringing both elbows down to the plinth and standing up again with all the weight on the hemiplegic leg (right hemiplegia)

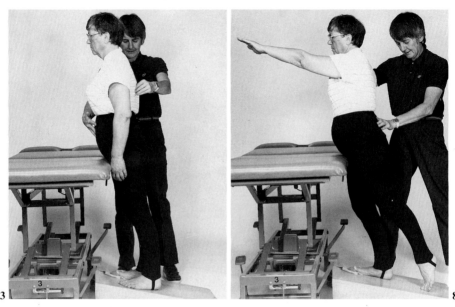

Fig. 8.13. Trunk and hip extension while standing on a wedge-shaped board, a rolled bandage placed beneath the affected toes (right hemiplegia)

Fig. 8.14. Standing on the sloping board with weight on the hemiplegic leg and the sound hand lifted from the plinth (right hemiplegia)

With his thighs against the plinth he takes a step backwards with his sound foot and leaves it resting with the big toe in contact with the supporting surface. He then raises his sound arm in front of him (Fig. 8.14).

First with his feet together and then with his sound foot behind him, the patient bends forwards until his elbows are resting on the plinth. With his hands clasped together and his forehead resting on them he returns to the upright position. Keeping his forehead in contact with his hands will ensure that he does not extend his neck in order to extend his trunk (Fig. 8.15 a–c). The therapist facilitates the movement by placing one of her arms around in front of his abdomen and guiding him upwards. She also helps him to keep his thighs in contact with the plinth as he repeats the movement.

The activity not only improves selective hip extension, but also reduces hypertonicity in the plantar flexors of the ankle to an amazing degree. It is an activity which can help the patient to be able to walk without requiring a brace or calliper to hold his foot in dorsal flexion.

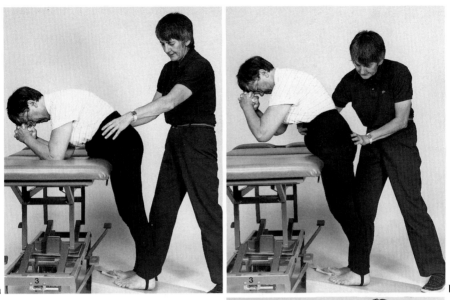

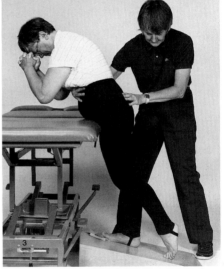

Fig. 8.15 a–c. Bringing both elbows down to the plinth and then standing upright again while standing on a wedge-shaped board (right hemiplegia). **a** The hips remain in contact with the plinth and the knees are extended. **b** The patient keeps her forehead in contact with her clasped hands. **c** The same movement with all the weight on the hemiplegic leg

8.2.5 Weight Bearing on the Hemiplegic Leg While Placing the Sound Foot on a Step

The patient stands on his hemiplegic leg and lifts his sound foot onto a step which is placed in front of him. The therapist stands at the patient's hemiplegic side with one hand assisting hip extension and the other resting on his opposite side, helping him to keep his weight towards her (Fig. 8.16a). The therapist as-

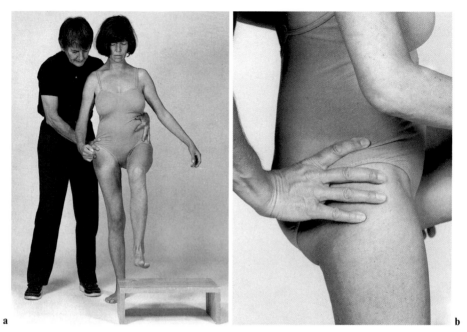

a   b

Fig. 8.16 a, b. Facilitating hip extension when the sound foot is placed on a low step (right hemiplegia). **a** The patient's knee points forwards over her foot. **b** The therapist assists extension and outward rotation of the hip

sists extension of the hemiplegic hip by placing her thumb over the head of the patient's femur and guiding it forwards with the appropriate amount of pressure. In other words, her hand acts as an accessory hip extensor, correcting the position of the pelvis over the femur and the femur over the foot (Fig. 8.16b). The patient is thus able to prevent his knee from snapping back into a hyperextended position. It would be impossible for the therapist's thumb alone to overcome the full force of the patient's extensor musculature pushing the knee backwards. Her hand only facilitates the correct movement as the patient tries to control the position of the knee himself, understanding what is required of him.

The patient places his foot lightly on the step and then returns it to the floor again. As his control improves he is asked to tap the foot repeatedly on the step without any movement taking place in the hemiplegic leg. He should be instructed to place the whole foot flat on the step and not just to make contact with his big toe, which requires far less activity. The number of times he taps the foot on the step concurrently is gradually increased.

Once the patient can perform the activity correctly and repeatedly, the height of the step in front of him can be increased (Fig. 8.17 a, b). Tapping his sound foot on the step demands more and more selective hip activity together with lower abdominal activity. The patient may have difficulty in stabilising his upper trunk while flexing his lower (Fig. 8.18 a). If he has learned to control his

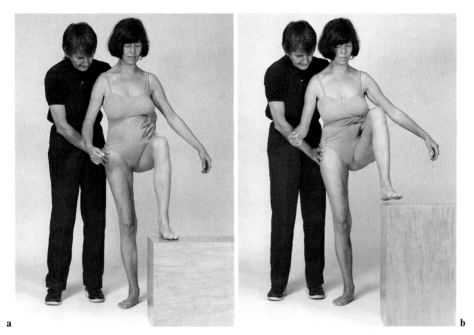

Fig. 8.17 a, b. Tapping the sound foot on a step. The height of the step is increased (right hemiplegia)

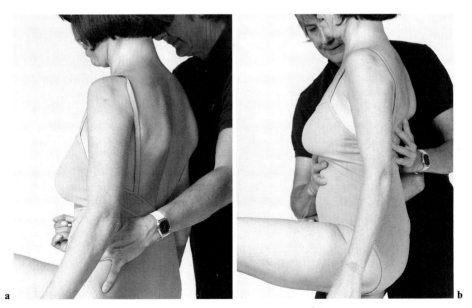

Fig. 8.18 a, b. Assisting extension of the thoracic spine when the sound leg is lifted (right hemiplegia). **a** Difficulty in stabilising the upper trunk. **b** The therapist supports the thorax

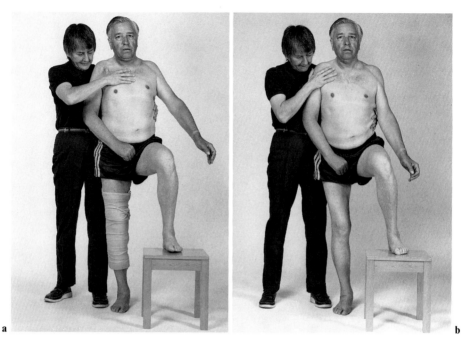

Fig. 8.19 a, b. Learning to extend the hemiplegic leg actively (right hemiplegia). **a** The knee extension splint enables the patient to experience taking weight through his affected leg. **b** Immediately afterwards he maintains the extension actively

hip without help, then the therapist can support his thorax, with one of her hands behind him at the appropriate level and the other on his lower rib cage in the front (Fig. 8.18 b).

N. B. On no account should the patient practise weight bearing on the hemiplegic leg with the knee hyperextended. Firstly, he would be practising an incorrect movement which may be difficult to correct later, and, secondly, spasticity in the plantar flexors of the ankle increases if the total extensor synergy is used.

If the patient is unable to maintain extension of his leg, due to disturbed sensation, hypotonus or spasticity in flexion, the activity can be practised with a splint holding his knee extended. The patient will often be able to repeat the movement without the splint directly afterwards when he has felt the movement, the tonus has been sufficiently increased or the flexor spasticity has been reduced through the weight bearing (Fig. 8.19 a, b).

To enable the patient to experience the movement of his knee during weight bearing, the therapist can give him total support and guide his leg into the correct positions. She stands beside the patient, places one of her legs behind his knee and her other in front of it and draws his body towards her. She uses one hand to help him lift his sound leg into the air (Fig. 8.20). By abducting and ad-

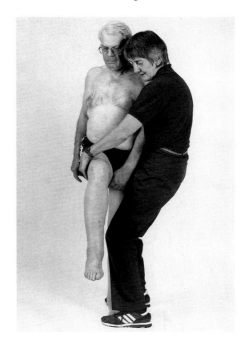

Fig. 8.20. Experiencing the movement of the knee while bearing weight on the hemiplegic leg. The therapist supports the patient's knee between her legs and helps him to hold his sound leg in the air (left hemiplegia)

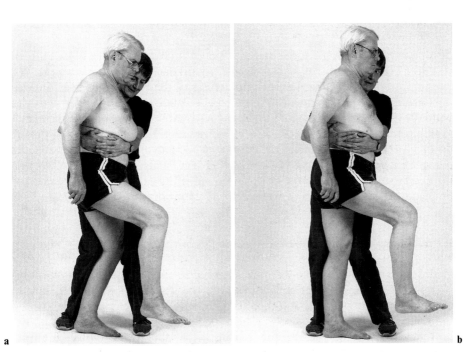

a   b

Fig. 8.21 a, b. Facilitating extensor activity in the hemiplegic knee while bearing weight. The therapist draws the patient's weight towards her, and by adducting and abducting her legs alternately she flexes and extends his knee slowly (left hemiplegia)

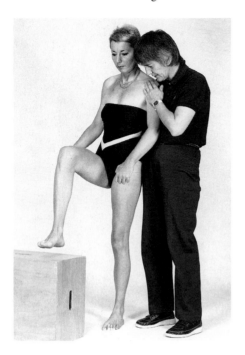

Fig. 8.22. Weight bearing on the hemiplegic leg with the sound foot placed first on one side of the step and then the other (left hemiplegia)

ducting her legs alternately, the therapist flexes and extends the patient's affected knee (Fig. 8.21a, b). Her hands clasped round his waist keep his weight well over his supporting leg and ensure elongation of the hemiplegic side. The patient should not place his sound foot on the step or perform other activities with it while being assisted in this way as he would then not perceive the activity in his hemiplegic leg. He is asked to assist actively in extending and flexing his hemiplegic knee as he feels the correct movement, and the therapist reduces the amount of support she is giving with her legs. When the patient can extend his knee without her help, the step can be put in front of him once again, and he places his sound foot on it while actively controlling his affected leg.

8.2.6 Weight Bearing on the Hemiplegic Leg with the Sound Leg Abducting

With some support from the therapist standing at his side, the patient places his sound foot on a raised step in front of him. He lifts it up and places it first to the lateral side of the step and then to the medial. As in the previous activity, the patient should place the sole of his foot flat on the step each time and not make contact with only his big toe (Fig. 8.22). The therapist can place the front of her hip behind the patient's hemiplegic hip, helping him to keep it forward in extension, while one of her hands maintains the correct position of his hemiplegic shoulder.

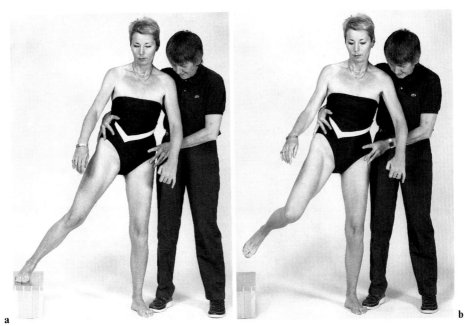

Fig. 8.23 a, b. Weight bearing on the hemiplegic leg with the sound leg abducting (left hemiplegia). **a** The patient places her sound foot on a step placed at her side, with her toes facing forwards. **b** The therapist assists hip extension

A step is placed some distance away on the patient's sound side. The therapist assists extension of the hemiplegic hip with one of her hands as he lifts his sound leg sideways to place it on the step. The therapist's other hand in his waist on the sound side maintains the patient's position with his weight well over his hemiplegic leg (Fig. 8.23 a). Increased selective extensor activity in the hip of the supporting leg is demanded if the patient places his sound foot on the step with the toes facing anteriorly and not laterally.

He lifts his sound foot off the step and holds it in the air above the step, while maintaining the position of his trunk and hemiplegic leg (Fig. 8.23 b). He then replaces his foot on the step and after repeating the movement a few times returns it to the ground.

When the patient can maintain the extension of his hemiplegic hip unaided while abducting his sound leg, the therapist can inhibit the associated reaction in flexion of the affected arm. She supports his extended, abducted arm with her chest. With one hand the therapist holds the patient's hand and fingers in dorsal extension and with her other in his waist on the sound side she keeps his weight over the affected leg (Fig. 8.24).

As the patient's control improves the therapist can use the hand that was in his waist beneath the hemiplegic shoulder to support the arm in abduction with outward rotation as the patient places his sound foot sideways on the step and brings it down to the floor again (Fig. 8.25).

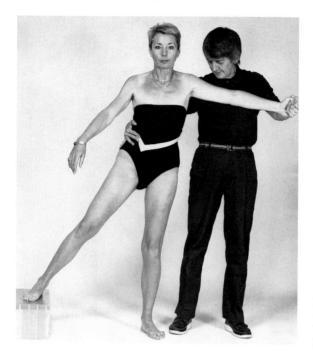

Fig. 8.24. Weight bearing on the hemiplegic leg with abduction of the hip. The therapist supports the patient's hemiplegic arm on her chest and keeps the weight over the affected side (left hemiplegia)

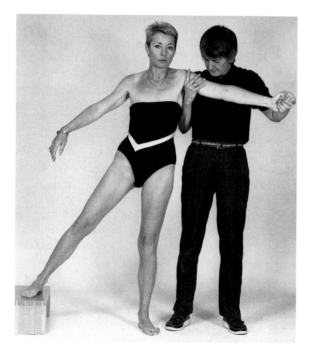

Fig. 8.25. Inhibiting flexor spasticity in the hemiplegic arm when the patient places her sound foot on a step at her side and tries to control her weight bearing hip unaided (left hemiplegia)

8.2.7 Hip Extension with Abduction and Outward Rotation

The patient stands with his back against a wall and then flexes both knees with his hips abducted and outwardly rotated. His back slides down the wall as his knees flex.

The therapist sits in front of the patient on a stool and with her knees and her hands presses his knees out sideways so that his hips are abducted and laterally rotated. The patient will often have difficulty keeping his back flat against the wall, and the loss of abduction during extensor activity of the hips will cause his feet to pronate (Fig. 8.26).

The therapist instructs him to tense his abdominal muscles and presses his knees more firmly away from each other (Fig. 8.27).

Keeping his entire back and his head against the wall the patient flexes his knees as far as he can and then extends them again. He tries to go down further each time as he repeats the movement (Fig. 8.28 a, b). The therapist uses her hands to press his knees firmly outwards so that they face over the long axes of his feet.

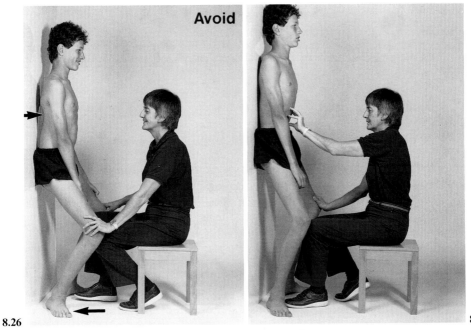

8.26   **8.27**

Fig. 8.26. Regaining active extension of the hip with abduction and outward rotation. The patient's back must remain flat against the wall and his knees point directly over his feet (right hemiplegia)

Fig. 8.27. Correcting the starting position, the therapist asks the patient to tense his abdominal muscles and presses his knees firmly away from each other (right hemiplegia)

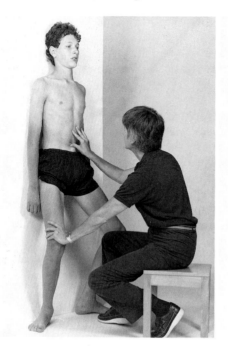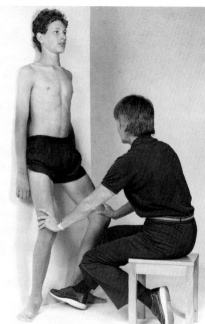

a   b

Fig. 8.28 a, b. Sliding down the wall with the hips abducted and outwardly rotated (right hemiplegia). **a** The therapist stimulates abdominal muscle activity as the patient flexes and extends his knees slowly. **b** She presses his knees away from one another so that they point over his feet

8.2.8 Active Plantar Flexion of the Ankles with Flexed Knees

Plantar flexion of the affected foot is first practised in sitting (Fig. 8.29) and standing (Fig. 8.30a, b), with the therapist guiding the correct movement. Then the patient stands facing a wall and supports himself slightly with his sound hand. He flexes his knees as he raises his heels off the ground simultaneously. The knees flex exactly the same amount as the feet plantarflex, so that the patient's head remains at the same level.

The patient will have difficulty at first in keeping his trunk extended as his knees flex. His hemiplegic foot will also tend to invert as he plantarflexes actively, and his toes will flex instead of extending (Fig. 8.31a). The therapist kneels beside the patient and with one hand over his thoracic spine helps him to maintain extension. She instructs him to tense his abdominal muscles at the same time. With her other hand she helps him to extend his toes (Fig. 8.31b).

The patient stabilises his trunk himself, and the therapist facilitates the correct movement of the hemiplegic foot, i. e. toes extended and foot not inverting (Fig. 8.32a). His heels should be held towards each other as they leave the floor, and his knees should point over his feet, and not medially.

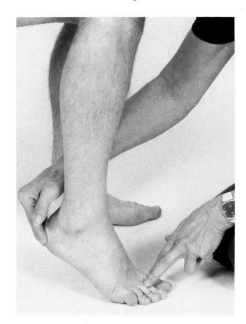

Fig. 8.29. Facilitating active plantar flexion of the hemiplegic foot without the toes flexing (right hemiplegia)

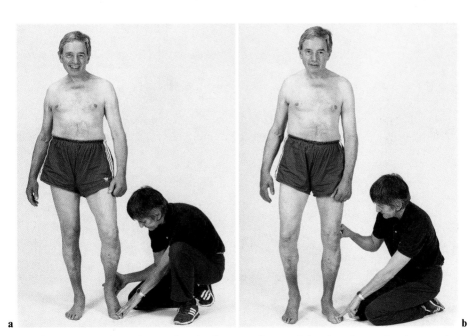

a

b

Fig. 8.30 a, b. Learning to plantarflex the foot selectively (left hemiplegia). **a** The therapist facilitates the correct movement. **b** The patient repeats the movement with his sound foot

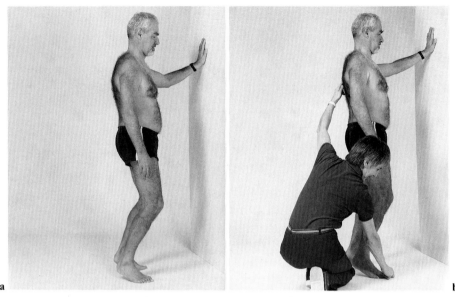

Fig. 8.31 a, b. Going up on the toes, with a wall for support (right hemiplegia). **a** The patient has difficulty in maintaining trunk extension and in preventing plantar inversion of the hemiplegic foot and flexion of the toes. **b** The therapist corrects the position of the trunk and foot

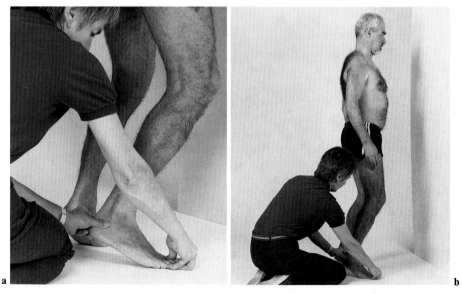

Fig. 8.32 a, b. Facilitating selective plantarflexion of the foot during weight bearing (right hemiplegia). **a** The therapist inhibits flexion of the toes and corrects the position of the ankle. **b** The patient holds the corrected position actively without the support of the wall

When the movement can be performed accurately with only a little support from the therapist, the patient removes his hand from the wall and tries to maintain his balance actively as he raises and lowers his heels (Fig. 8.32 b).

8.2.9 Controlling the Hemiplegic Leg Actively Against Gravity

The patient stands with the plinth behind him, and the therapist, kneeling in front of him, lifts his hemiplegic leg into flexion. Without supporting himself against the plinth, the patient controls his leg actively as the therapist guides it down towards the floor. The patient must eventually be able to let his foot rest on the floor without any weight on it, nor any unwanted activity occurring in the foot. Only when he is able to control his leg in this way will he be able to swing his leg forward while walking.

At first the patient leans against the plinth behind him to reduce the demand for balance when the therapist lifts his leg to about 90° flexion of the hip and knee. The therapist sits on a stool in front of him, flexes his leg and then asks the patient to hold its weight as she lowers it slowly to the ground without his losing control and pushing the foot against the floor (Fig. 8.33 a, b). Most patients will have difficulty in transferring weight adequately over the sound leg while keeping the trunk extended.

When he can control his leg throughout its range of movement with his but-

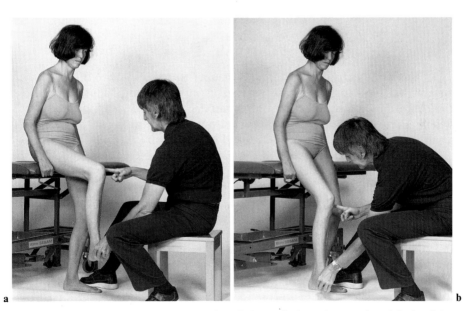

Fig. 8.33 a, b. Learning to control the hemiplegic leg actively against gravity (right hemiplegia). **a** At first the patient leans against a plinth. **b** She tries to lower her foot slowly to the floor

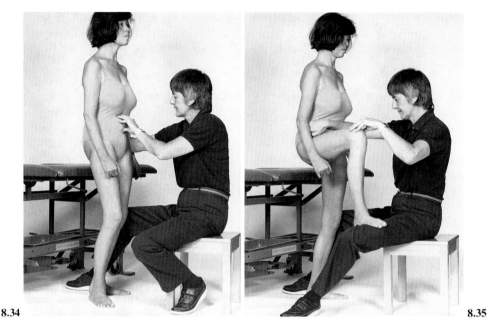

8.34   8.35

Fig. 8.34. Transferring weight over the sound leg without the support of the plinth, and relaxing the hemiplegic leg (right hemiplegia)

Fig. 8.35. Standing on the sound leg with the hemiplegic foot supported on the therapist's knee (right hemiplegia)

tocks supported against the plinth, the patient stands upright and transfers his weight over his sound leg. The therapist sits on a stool at first, so that she can use one of her legs placed beside his sound leg to give him support and confidence. The patient maintains firm pressure with his leg against the therapist's as she corrects the posture of his trunk (Fig. 8.34).

Keeping his sound leg against the therapist's leg the patient assists as she lifts his hemiplegic leg into the air and places his foot on her other thigh. The therapist corrects the patient's position, particularly the too active elevation of his pelvis on the hemiplegic side until he can let his leg stay quietly supported without over-activity and with his trunk erect (Fig. 8.35).

The therapist holds the patient's toes in dorsal extension and asks him to hold the weight of his leg actively as she guides it towards the ground. He tries not to push his foot down as it nears the floor. Should the patient hitch the side of his pelvis up as he maintains control of his leg through eccentric flexor activity, the therapist places her free hand over his iliac crest on that side and instructs him to let it remain in a neutral position (Fig. 8.36a, b). As his control improves, the therapist kneels as she guides his foot down to the floor (Fig. 8.37).

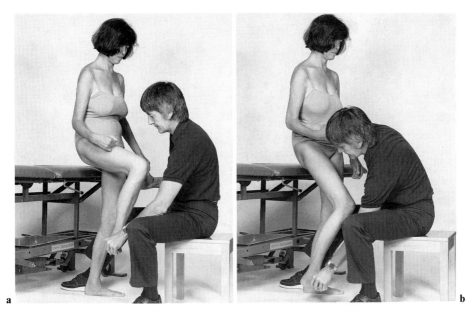

a   b

Fig. 8.36 a, b. Controlling the hemiplegic leg actively against gravity (right hemiplegia). **a** The therapist holds the patient's toes in dorsal extension and asks her to hold the weight of her leg. **b** The side of the pelvis is not hitched up, despite the flexor activity of the leg

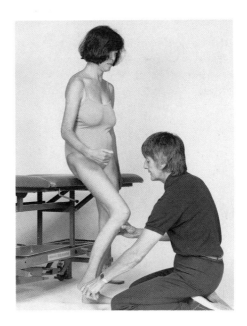

Fig. 8.37. Controlling the hemiplegic leg actively with minimal help, until the foot rests lightly on the floor (right hemiplegia)

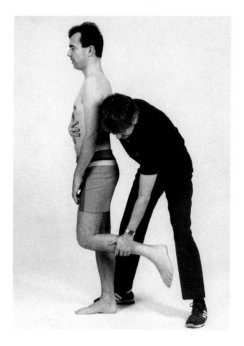

Fig. 8.38. Supporting the patient while lifting his hemiplegic foot off the floor behind him. The therapist places one hand over the patient's chest anteriorly (left hemiplegia)

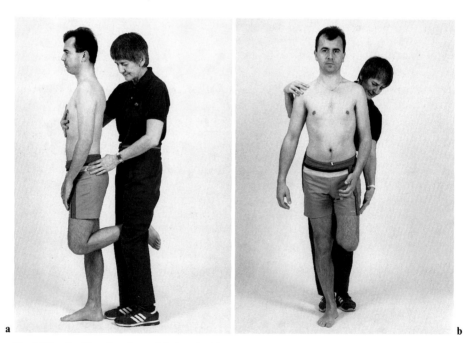

Fig. 8.39 a, b. Keeping the pelvis level while standing on the sound leg (left hemiplegia). **a** The therapist holds the patient's hemiplegic foot between her knees. **b** The patient relaxes his leg and prevents the hip from abducting

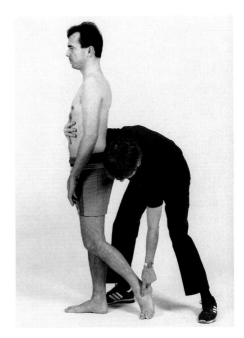

Fig. 8.40. Lowering the hemiplegic foot slowly to rest on the floor behind (left hemiplegia)

8.2.10 Active Control of the Hemiplegic Leg when the Hip Is Extended

When walking the patient will also need to control his hemiplegic leg when it is behind him with the hip extended, as it will be at the beginning of the swing phase. Walking backwards requires the ability to flex the knee while extending the hip actively.

The therapist stands behind the patient and lifts his hemiplegic leg from the floor. To help him maintain his balance confidently when doing so, she should place her other hand around his sound side and support his trunk from the front (Fig. 8.38).

She places the shin of his hemiplegic leg between her legs and holds it there as she adjusts the level of the patient's pelvis (Fig. 8.39 a). She reduces her support until she is only holding his shoulder or the sides of his pelvis (Fig. 8.39 b).

Once the patient is balancing in the position, the therapist takes his hemiplegic foot in her hand and slowly lowers it to the floor, asking him to control the movement actively as she does so. The therapist brings the patient's foot to rest on the floor behind him, and he maintains his balance while relaxing his foot and letting it remain there (Fig. 8.40).

The side flexors of the trunk must work hard to maintain the level of the pelvis from above, as otherwise the leg would need to support it actively from below.

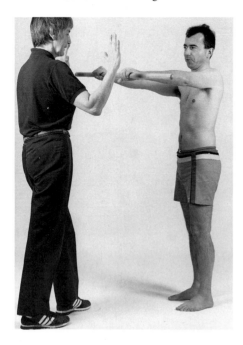

Fig. 8.41. Giving quick approximating taps to the pole stimulates abdominal muscle activity (left hemiplegia)

8.2.11 Moving the Arms Actively While Standing

Activities which involve moving the arms while in a standing position will stimulate trunk activity and will also help the patient to become accustomed to the upright position without being afraid. The patient will also enjoy the activities.

8.2.11.1 Holding a Pole in Both Hands

The patient grasps a pole with both his hands and holds it in front of him. The therapist gives quick approximating taps against the pole and instructs the patient to maintain his balance as she does so (Fig. 8.41). The patient's abdominal muscles are activated by the brisk thump of the therapist's hand contacting the pole. The therapist can change her position from one side to the other to activate the desired muscles.

8.2.11.2 Hitting a Ball with a Pole

The patient stands with his knees slightly flexed. A third person throws a hard ball which the patient hits away with the pole held horizontally in both his hands. The therapist, standing at the patient's hemiplegic side keeps his weight evenly distributed over both his legs and can help hold his hemiplegic hand firmly on the pole.

The patient keeps his arms extended and hits the ball back to the person throwing it (Fig. 8.42). The activity in his trunk is that of extension.

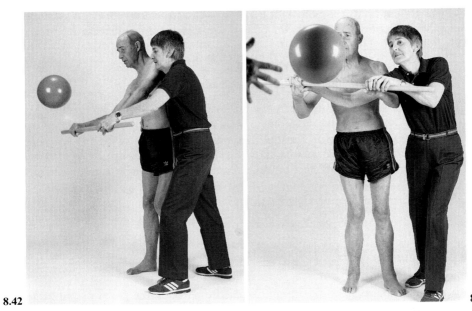

Fig. 8.42. Hitting a ball with a pole held horizontally in both hands (left hemiplegia)

Fig. 8.43. Holding the pole with flexed elbows and then hitting the ball away (left hemiplegia)

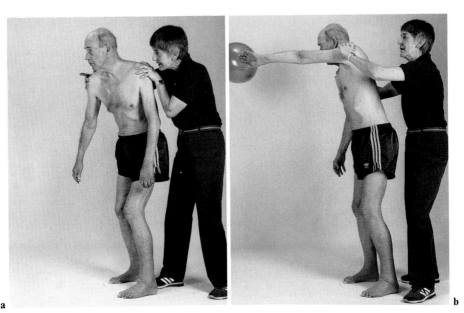

a

b

Fig. 8.44 a, b. Hitting a balloon away with the hemiplegic hand (left hemiplegia). **a** The therapist rotates the hemiplegic side well back. **b** The patient lets his arm swing forward without lifting the hand itself

The patient holds the pole with his elbows flexed and hits the ball away by extending his elbows. Abdominal activity is stimulated to stabilise his trunk (Fig. 8.43).

8.2.11.3 Hitting a Balloon Away with the Hemiplegic Hand

The therapist stands beside the patient with one of her hands on each of his shoulders. She rotates his hemiplegic side well back, and as a third person throws the balloon towards him the therapist helps him to swing his arm and the trunk side forwards so that his hand hits the balloon. The patient is told not to try to lift his hand actively, but to let is swing forwards as if it were a tennis racquet. By so doing the arm moves forwards in a normal way and is not flexed in the total flexion synergy (Fig. 8.44a, b).

8.3 Conclusion

Correct, confident standing will automatically improve the patient's ability to walk more normally. Most patients will have difficulty transferring their weight over to the sound side as well as to the hemiplegic side. Standing on one leg requires considerable trunk activity as the pelvis on the side of the leg which is no longer on the ground has to be suspended from above. Careful practice of the individual components of gait will improve the walking pattern far more than practising walking itself.

9 Ball Activities

Carefully chosen activities using a gymnastic ball can form a useful part of the treatment programme. A ball with its characteristic shape and movements is something very familiar to us all, an object which we have experienced since our earliest childhood. During the development of adult motor patterns, most people have at some time sat on a ball, lain on a ball, thrown, caught, bounced and kicked a ball. The experience can therefore be said to have formed an integral part of our motor learning. Even in countries where a ball as we know it is not available, children have had similar experiences using other round objects such as tree trunks, rolling stones or bound-up hides. The ball can be beneficial for the treatment for several reasons.

Patients of all ages enjoy the activities. They introduce variety and an element of fun into what can become a somewhat dull routine. Every day, or even twice a day the patient is expected to practise a series of activities to enable him to stand, walk or control his arm. Because of the long-term nature of the rehabilitation, such activities will be practised many times, and the variation which the ball affords will be much appreciated by the therapist as well as the patient.

The ball provides the patient with information from his surroundings, helping him to carry out the movement correctly.

- The patient is able to achieve a new skill which he can observe for himself and is not dependent upon the therapist telling him that the movement was a "little better". The successful accomplishment is a positive experience for him.
- The way in which the ball moves, or does not move, enables the therapist to observe compensatory activity more easily.
- The ball supports the weight of a part of the body, and the desired muscles can be activated without so much effort, even when the patient is still not able to move independently.
- Subtle and highly co-ordinated muscle activity can be stimulated when working with patients who are functioning at a very high level.

The use of the ball has been advocated in many different treatment concepts. The activities which have been selected for this chapter are those which have proved to be particularly useful for many patients with hemiplegia.

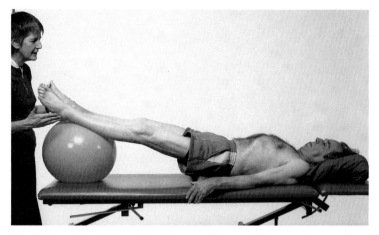

Fig. 9.1. Lifting both buttocks off the plinth with both knees extended (left hemiplegia)

Muscle activity is stimulated in three different ways:

1. The patient moves the ball in a specific direction.
2. The patient maintains a certain position and prevents movement of the ball.
3. The ball moves or is moved and the patient reacts.

The resulting muscle activity still adheres to the principles of the tentacle and the bridge as described in Chap. 2. The *tentacle* is that part of the body which moves in space from the part supported on the ball. The *bridge* is the part or parts of the body supported between the ball and the floor (Klein-Vogelbach 1990). The size of the ball is very important for activities where the patient sits or lies with his whole weight supported on the ball. When sitting on the ball, the vertical distance between the patient's hip joint and the floor must be at least the same, if not a bit greater than the distance from his knee joint to the floor. The ball should be pumped up firmly enough so that when the patient's weight is on it, its contour is only moderately flattened, still allowing a free rolling movement.

9.1 Ball Activities in Supine Lying

The patient lies on his back with both his feet supported on a ball. He raises his buttocks off the supporting surface and does not allow the ball to move at all.

When the patient is not yet able to get down on to the floor, the activity is practised while lying on a plinth. The therapist helps the patient to put both his legs on the ball which is placed directly in line with the long axis of his body. The activity is easier if the ball is placed nearer to the patient's knees at first.

The patient's arms remain at his sides as he straightens his knees by pressing the ball away from him and lifts his buttocks off the plinth. Both knees re-

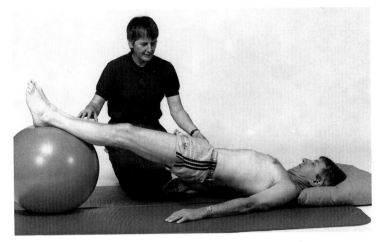

Fig. 9.2. Holding the ball in the same position when the buttocks are lifted off the mat (right hemiplegia)

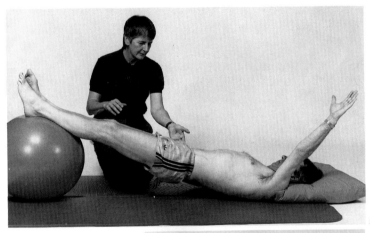

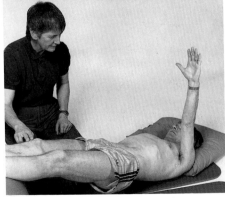

Fig. 9.3 a, b. Using trunk activity to prevent the ball from moving when the sound arm is lifted. The pelvis stays level (right hemiplegia)

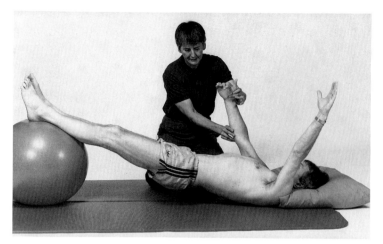

Fig. 9.4. Maintaining the position of the ball when the hemiplegic arm is moved passively without any resistance to the movement (right hemiplegia)

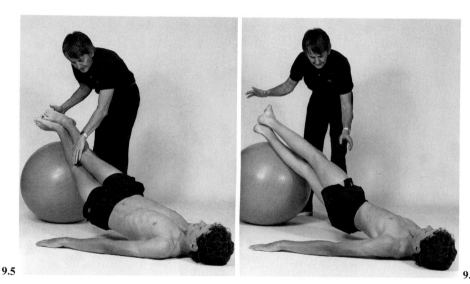

9.5

9.6

Fig. 9.5. Turning both legs towards the sound side with the seat raised from the supporting surface (right hemiplegia)

Fig. 9.6. Holding the ball steady when both legs are turned to the hemiplegic side (right hemiplegia)

main in an extended position and the patient tries to keep the ball completely stationary (Fig. 9.1). Should the ball move, the therapist assists by guiding the patient's legs appropriately, so that he can feel the correction. She should not hold the ball as the patient would be unaware that he was being assisted. The same activity can be carried out with the patient lying on a firm rubber mat on the floor (Fig. 9.2). As the patient's control improves, the ball is placed gradually further and further away from him until it is beneath his heels. The trunk side flexors work actively to prevent the ball from moving sideways.

The patient is asked to raise his sound arm to about 90° flexion at the shoulder. The amount of trunk activity is increased when his arm is not pressing against the floor to stabilise the ball (Fig. 9.3 a, b).

Should the patient have sufficient active movement in his hemiplegic arm, he raises it as well and holds it in position parallel to his sound arm. If the arm is paralysed, the therapist holds it in extension and moves it into elevation and back again, asking the patient to allow the movement without resistance in any direction (Fig. 9.4).

When the patient has regained sufficient control of his trunk, i. e. can hold the ball stationary without the use of his arms, he is asked to turn his legs to one side until the lateral border of the underneath leg is in contact with the ball. The other leg lies supported on the leg below, and the patient tries not to let his pelvis sag towards the floor (Fig. 9.5).

He learns to carry out the activity towards both sides and still maintain his pelvis in line with his body. The therapist removes her hands and the patient holds the ball steady. Both his arms remain flat on the floor beside him (Fig. 9.6).

9.1.1 Lifting the Ball off the Bed with Both Legs

The patient lies supine and places both legs over the top of the ball. He draws the ball towards him, presses his heels against it and lifts it up. His hips and

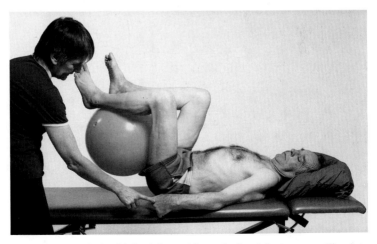

Fig. 9.7. Lifting the ball off the plinth with both legs without the hemiplegic arm pulling into flexion (left hemiplegia)

knees flex actively, and he lifts his buttocks off the bed as well. His spine remains flat on the bed.

The activity can be carried out on a plinth at first. The therapist helps the
patient to hold the ball in place and to keep his hemiplegic arm lying on the
plinth at his side (Fig. 9.7).

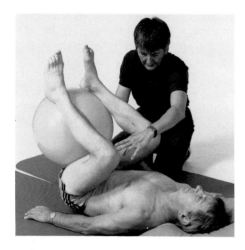

Fig. 9.8. Keeping the knees level and
apart when the ball is lifted (left hemiplegia)

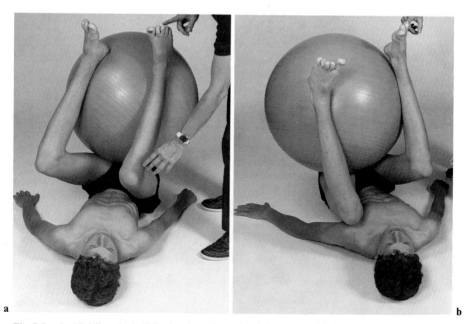

a   b

Fig. 9.9 a, b. Holding the ball in the air and moving it from one side to the other with selective
lateral flexion of the lumbar spine (right hemiplegia). **a** To the hemiplegic side. **b** To the
sound side

The patient learns to keep both knees apart and at the same level as he lifts his buttocks off the floor by tensing his lower abdominal muscles (Fig. 9.8). He keeps his back and his shoulders flat on the floor despite the lower trunk flexion.

When he can lift the ball correctly, the patient moves it first to one side and

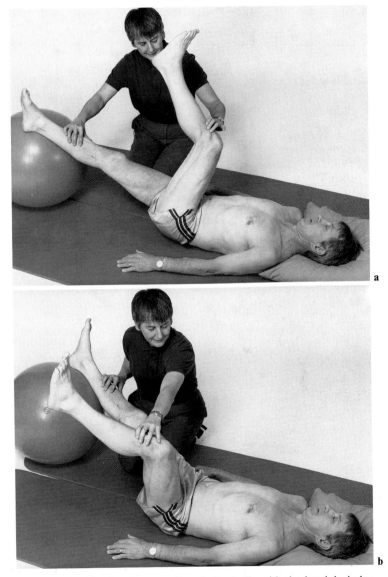

Fig. 9.10 a, b. Abducting and adducting the sound leg rhythmically with the hemiplegic leg supported on a ball (right hemiplegia)

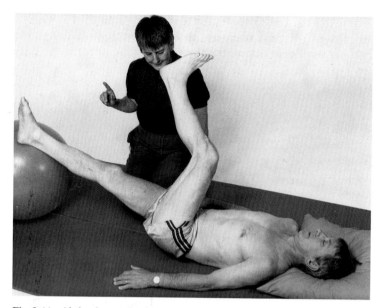

Fig. 9.11. Abducting and adducting the sound leg with the hip flexed to 90°. The other leg moves reactively in the contralateral direction (right hemiplegia)

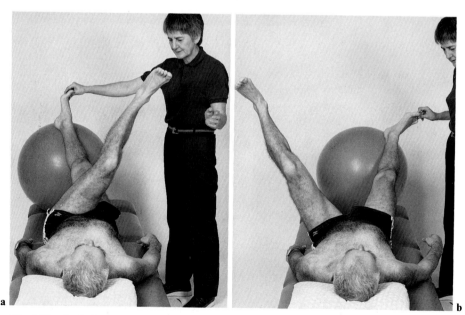

Fig. 9.12 a, b. Lying on a plinth with the sound leg abducting and adducting and the upper trunk stabilised (right hemiplegia)

then to the other with his back still remaining flat on the floor. He uses his trunk side flexors selectively to move the ball, his hips and knees remaining in the same position relative to each other throughout the movement (Fig. 9.9 a, b).

The flexor activity required to lift the ball can be alternated with the extensor activity used to raise the patient's seat off the plinth as described in the previous sequence (Fig. 9.3).

9.1.2 Abducting and Adducting One Leg with the Other Leg Supported on the Ball

The patient lies with one of his legs supported on the ball. He lifts his other leg until the hip is flexed to at least 90° and moves it rhythmically from one side to the other by adducting and abducting his hip. The ball with the leg supported on it moves reactively in the contralateral direction.

The patient's trunk and head lie supported. His arms are in an abducted position and remain in contact with the floor, the palms of his hands facing downwards. The therapist helps him to place his hemiplegic leg on the ball in a relaxed position, and he lifts his sound foot into the air. Maintaining an angle of more than 90° of hip flexion, he adducts the sound leg, allowing his hemiplegic leg to move with the ball in the contralateral direction (Fig. 9.10a).

With one of her hands on each of his legs, the therapist assists the movement as the patient swings his sound leg towards abduction, his hemiplegic leg abducting simultaneously (Fig. 9.10b).

The patient repeats the movement rhythmically and easily from abduction to adduction, and the therapist assists the movement less and less until he is moving on his own (Fig. 9.11).

The activity can also be carried out when the patient is lying on a plinth (Fig. 9.12a, b).

When the movement can be performed easily, the patient raises his sound arm to about 90° of flexion of the shoulder. If he has some voluntary movement in his hemiplegic arm he can hold a pole horizontally in both hands (Fig. 9.13). The stabilisation of his trunk becomes more active without the help of his sound arm pressing against the floor. The patient who is able to control his hemiplegic arm more actively holds it vertically, parallel to the sound arm, as he moves his legs. He will at first have difficulty in holding his arm in position (Fig. 9.14a). The therapist helps him to keep the arm in the correct position and gradually reduces the amount of support (Fig. 9.14b).

The same activity can be practised with the sound leg resting on the ball and the hemiplegic leg moving from adduction to abduction, but will be far more difficult for the patient to control (Fig. 9.15).

He will probably need to reduce the speed of the movement and leave his sound arm on the floor beside him. The therapist assists the movement of both legs, as necessary (Fig. 9.16a, b).

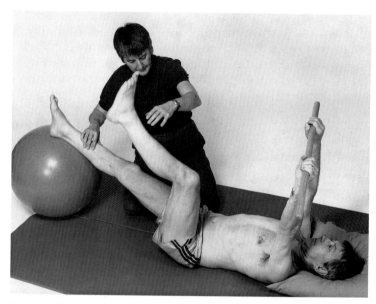

Fig. 9.13. Holding a pole horizontally in both hands while the sound leg moves (right hemiplegia)

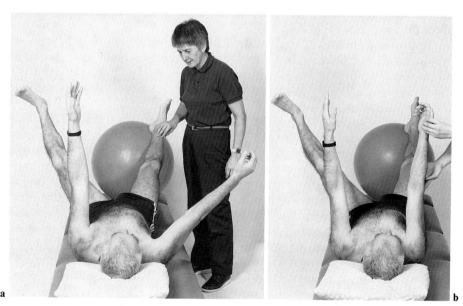

a   b

Fig. 9.14 a, b. Holding both arms vertical and parallel to one another while the legs abduct and adduct (right hemiplegia). **a** The patient has difficulty in keeping his hemiplegic arm in position. **b** The therapist corrects the position of the arm

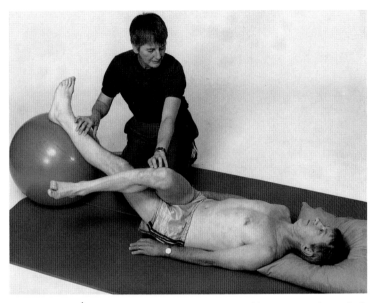

Fig. 9.15. Abducting and adducting the hemiplegic leg with the sound leg supported on a ball. The therapist facilitates the rhythmical movement (right hemiplegia)

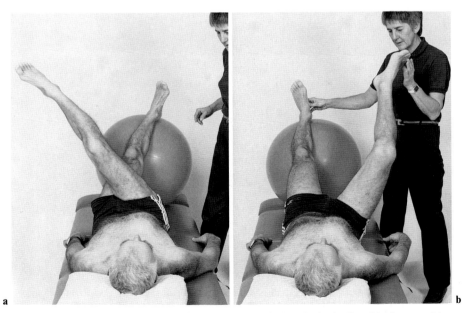

a   b

Fig. 9.16 a, b. Abducting and adducting the hemiplegic leg rhythmically with the sound leg moving in the contralateral direction (right hemiplegia)

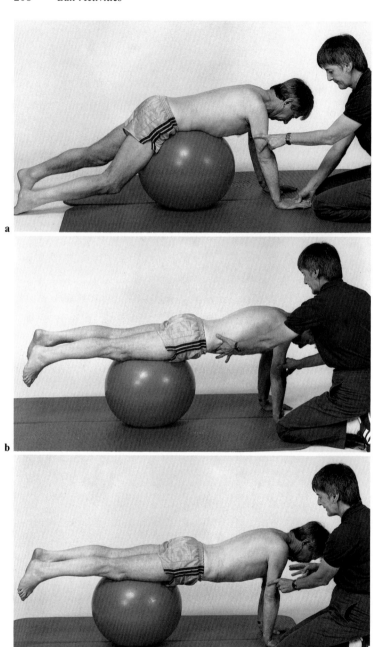

Fig. 9.17 a–c. Lying prone on the ball with weight taken through both arms (right hemiplegia). **a** From a kneeling position the patient lies on the ball and the therapist places his hemiplegic hand flat on the floor. **b** He brings his weight forwards and holds his trunk in a straight line. **c** He holds the ball steady with his legs extended and adducted

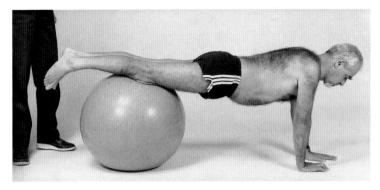

Fig. 9.18. More abdominal muscle activity is required when the hands are placed further away from the ball (right hemiplegia)

9.2 Ball Activities in Prone Lying

9.2.1 Lying Prone on the Ball with Weight Supported Through Both Arms

From a kneeling position on the floor, the patient lies over the ball in front of him. The therapist helps him to place his hemiplegic hand flat on the floor and to maintain extension of the elbow as he brings his weight forwards (Fig. 9.17 a).

The patient brings his weight further forward until his feet leave the floor. He holds his legs extended and adducted and tries to maintain his trunk in a straight line without his abdomen sagging (Fig. 9.17 b).

More active control of the abdominal muscles is demanded when the patient's hands are placed further forwards, and the ball supports his weight more distally beneath his knees (Fig. 9.17 c). The patient should try to keep his thoracic spine extended, despite the considerable activity in the abdominal muscles.

With the therapist guiding his hemiplegic hand, the patient returns to a kneeling position with the ball in front of him.

As his ability improves, the patient learns to carry out the activity with less and less help from the therapist, until he can move forwards and maintain the position himself with his weight taken through both arms and only his knees in contact with the ball (Fig. 9.18).

9.2.2 Lower Trunk and Hip Flexion with Both Knees Supported on the Ball

When the patient is able to maintain the position in prone on the ball and can take weight confidently through his arms without the therapist assisting elbow extension, he can flex both his legs, drawing the ball towards his arms with his knees.

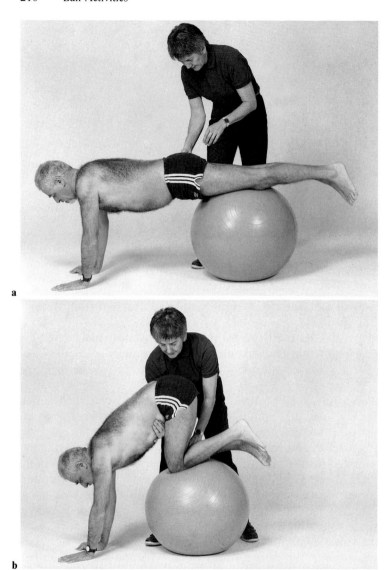

Fig. 9.19 a, b. Flexing the lower trunk with both knees supported on the ball. The therapist facilitates flexion of the lumbar spine and helps the patient to flex his hemiplegic leg (right hemiplegia)

The therapist places one hand beneath his lower abdomen to assist flexion of the lumbar spine and with her other hand helps the patient to flex his hemiplegic leg. Standing at his side she also enables the patient to maintain his balance (Fig. 9.19 a, b).

Once his hips and knees are flexed, the therapist places one hand on either

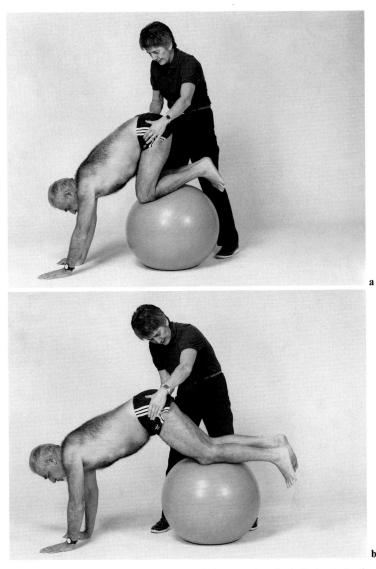

Fig. 9.20 a, b. Maintaining balance with less assistance and then moving the ball slowly back to the starting position (right hemiplegia)

side of the patient's pelvis and asks him to try to keep his balance as she gives less help (Fig. 9.20a).

The patient moves the ball away from his arms again to return to the starting position. The more slowly he allows the ball to move, the greater the amount of abdominal muscle activity (Fig. 9.20b). He can try to stop in a position on the way and hold the ball still. The movement sequence requires not

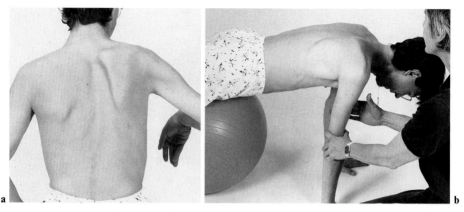

Fig. 9.21 a, b. Holding the ball still requires co-ordinated stabilisation from the trunk side flexors and the muscles around the shoulder (right hemiplegia)

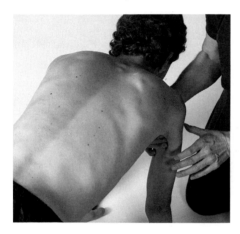

Fig. 9.22. Stimulating activity in the muscles which stabilise the scapulae on the chest wall (compare with Fig. 9.30 a, b; right hemiplegia)

only considerable lower trunk activity, but also co-ordinated stabilisation from the trunk side flexors to prevent the ball from moving sideways and to maintain balance.

It also stimulates activity in the muscles which stabilise the scapulae on the chest wall as well as in all the muscles acting on the shoulder (Fig. 9.21 a, b, 9.22).

9.2.3 Rotating the Trunk Until Only One Trochanter Is Supported on the Ball

More advanced patients can move from the prone position, rotating their trunk until only one of their hips is supported on the ball.

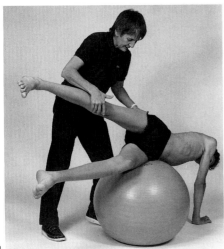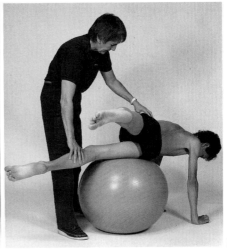

Fig. 9.23 a, b. Rotating the trunk until only one trochanter is supported on the ball. The therapist helps to extend and abduct the uppermost leg (right hemiplegia)

The patient moves the ball towards one side, rotating his trunk as he does so, the leg which is underneath moving forwards on the ball, the other leg abducting and extending in the air (Fig. 9.23 a). The movement is started with the ball beneath the patient's thighs and hips.

The therapist helps the patient to abduct and extend his uppermost leg and to control the movement of the ball.

The activity is carried out towards both sides, with the therapist giving less and less support until the patient can hold the ball in position on his own (Fig. 9.23 b).

9.3 Ball Activities in Sitting

The correct starting position is important before the ball is moved in any direction. The patient should be able to return to the exact position quickly and easily at any time. To sit quite still in the correct position on the ball in itself demands constant and co-ordinated activity from the muscles of the trunk.

The patient sits on the ball so that his seat is directly over its centre. His trunk is upright and in line with the diameter of the ball. His legs are slightly abducted, with his knees over his feet, i. e. his thighs in line with his feet. His hips and knees form right angles.

The therapist stands behind the patient to adjust his position, to give him adequate support and to control the ball with her legs if necessary (Fig. 9.24).

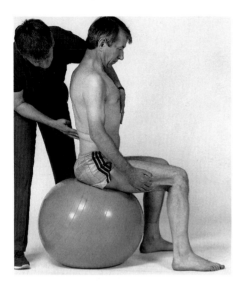

Fig. 9.24. Sitting upright on the ball with the lumbar spine extended (right hemiplegia)

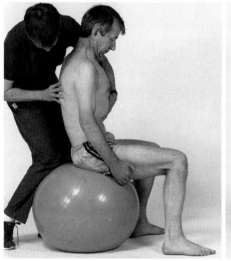

a

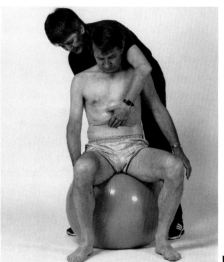

b

Fig. 9.25 a, b. Flexing the lumbar spine (right hemiplegia). **a** The therapist helps to stabilise the thoracic spine and moves the ball forwards with her knee. **b** The patient draws the ball forwards between his thighs

9.3.1 Flexing and Extending the Lumbar Spine

The patient draws the ball forwards between his legs while maintaining extension of his thoracic spine.

The therapist helps to stabilise the thorax, using one of her arms supporting the front of his chest and her other hand assisting extension from behind. With

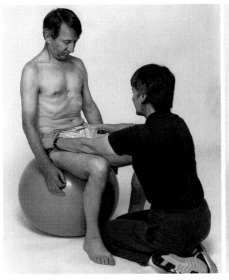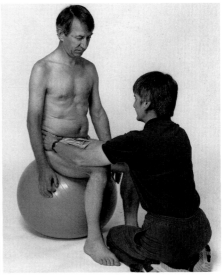

a   b

Fig. 9.26 a, b. Flexing and extending the lumbar spine. The therapist facilitates the movement of the pelvis (right hemiplegia)

one of her legs she moves the ball forwards in the required direction (Fig. 9.25 a).

Both the patient's hips remain in the same position of abduction and he tries to bring the ball forwards in the middle (Fig. 9.25 b).

When the patient requires less support the therapist can kneel in front of him and facilitate the movement with her hands placed over the sides of his pelvis. She can assist abduction of his hips with her elbows against the inside of his thighs (Fig. 9.26 a). The patient alternates the movement of the ball forwards by moving it backwards as far as he can so that his lumbar spine extends selectively (Fig. 9.26 b).

9.3.2 Lateral Flexion of the Lumbar Spine

Isolated lateral flexion of the lumbar spine is rather more difficult for the patient.

The therapist stands beside the patient and uses her arms to stabilise his thorax and take some of the weight of his trunk. She uses one of her knees to move the ball to the other side and the patient moves it back to the centre (Fig. 9.27).

The therapist stands on the other side of the patient and repeats the movement to the opposite side. From her position she can observe the spine directly and see if the movement is occurring in the lumbar region or not (Fig. 9.28).

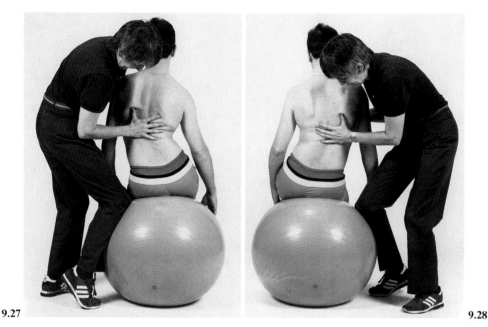

9.27   9.28

Fig. 9.27. Selective lateral flexion of the lumbar spine. The therapist helps to stabilise the thoracic spine and moves the ball towards the sound side with her knee (left hemiplegia)

Fig. 9.28. Stabilising the thoracic spine and moving the ball towards the hemiplegic side (left hemiplegia)

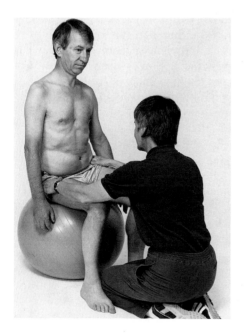

Fig. 9.29. Selective lateral flexion of the trunk with facilitation from the pelvis (right hemiplegia)

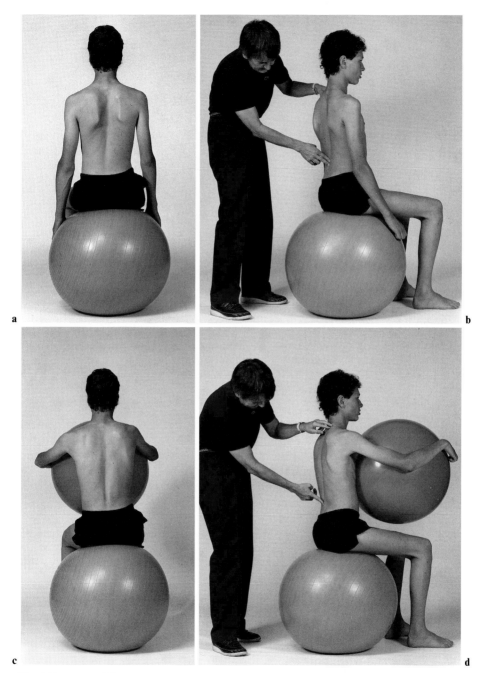

Fig. 9.30 a–d. Holding a ball in both arms to correct the position of the thoracic spine and scapulae (right hemiplegia). **a** Winging of the scapulae. **b** Over-active extension of the thoracic spine. **c** Scapulae in corrected position. **d** Normal kyphosis of the thoracic spine

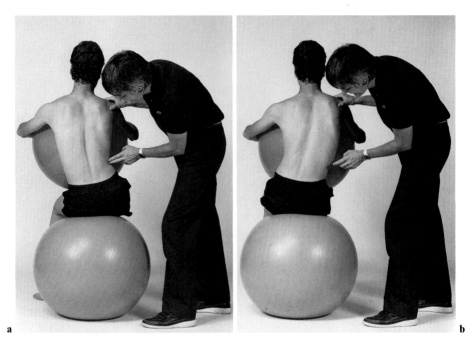

a   b

Fig. 9.31 a, b. Moving the ball from one side to the other and trying to localise the movement to the lumbar spine (right hemiplegia)

The patient participates increasingly actively as he feels the movement of the ball. The therapist reduces her assistance as he takes over the movement and uses her hands as required.

Eventually she can kneel in front of the patient and facilitate the movement of the pelvis with her hands, one on either side (Fig. 9.29).

The patient will often extend his spine too much in the thoracic region and his scapulae will no longer lie on the thoracic wall but assume a winged position (Fig. 9.30a, b).

Placing his arms round a ball which he holds against his chest can help to restore the normal kyphosis of the thoracic spine and correct the position of the scapulae (Fig. 9.30c, d). Holding the ball in his arms without effort, the patient can then move the ball on which he is sitting from one side to the other, trying to localise the movement to his lumbar spine with the help of the therapist. His shoulders should remain level (Fig. 9.31a, b).

9.3.3 Bouncing on the Ball

Stabilising his trunk in an upright position, the patient bounces on the ball by extending his knees selectively and then relaxing them again. His feet remain flat on the floor and his knees continue to point over his feet, moving neither

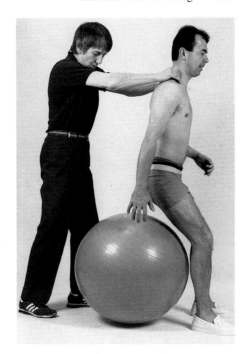

Fig. 9.32. Bouncing on the ball with the feet remaining flat on the floor and the lumbar spine extended (left hemiplegia)

towards nor away from one another. As his ability to maintain his balance improves, he can let his buttocks leave the ball after every third bounce and then return to contact it again and continue bouncing (Fig. 9.32).

9.3.4 Walking Both Feet Forwards Until Only the Shoulders Are Supported on the Ball

From a sitting position on the ball, the patient walks his feet forwards, step by step and rhythmically, until the ball is approximately beneath his scapulae and his feet underneath his knees. The patient tries to keep his trunk and thighs level, without allowing his seat to sag downwards (Fig. 9.33 a–c).

The therapist holds the patient's foot in a plantigrade position and prevents the toes from flexing or the foot from supinating, as they will tend to do. With her other hand she facilitates the movement from the patient's knee. The closer together the feet are, the more difficult it becomes to prevent the sideways movement of the ball. The hips should not abduct; the thighs should remain parallel to the line of the feet.

When the patient can maintain the position of his pelvis unaided and his hemiplegic foot remains flat on the floor, the therapist stands beside him and holds his arms parallel to one another at 90° flexion of the shoulder and with the elbows extended.

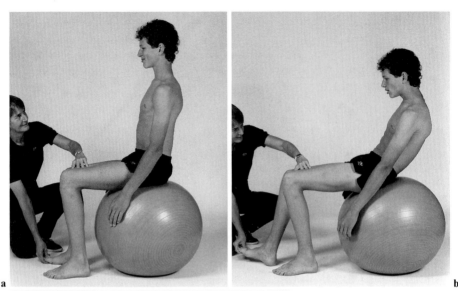

a   b

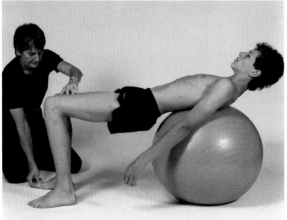

c

Fig. 9.33 a–c. Walking both feet forwards until only the shoulders are supported on the ball (right hemiplegia). **a** The therapist inhibits supination of the foot and flexion of the toes. **b** The patient moves his feet forwards, step by step. **c** He keeps his trunk and thighs level

The patient rotates his trunk forwards on one side, moving the ball towards that side and making the corresponding arm move towards the ceiling.

The therapist facilitates the movement by helping the patient lift one arm and by pushing downwards lightly on the other (Fig. 9.34a, b). The movement is repeated rhythmically from one side to the other. It is a difficult activity requiring selective trunk and leg control and only advanced patients will be able to do it.

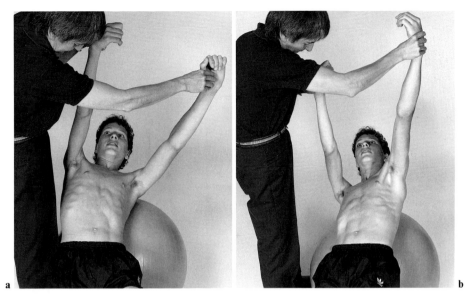

a   b

Fig. 9.34 a, b. Rotating the trunk and moving the ball from one side to the other. The therapist holds the arms in extension and facilitates the movement (right hemiplegia)

9.4 Ball Activities in Standing

9.4.1 Standing on One Leg with the Other Foot on a Moving Ball

The patient holds a pole horizontally in front of him, with his hands shoulder width apart. The therapist supports his hemiplegic hand with her hand placed over it and maintains dorsal flexion of his wrist. Her other hand holds his sound hand lightly on the pole.

The patient stands on his hemiplegic leg and places his sound foot on a large ball in front of him. He must do so without hyper-extending the affected knee.

The therapist stands facing the patient and also places her foot on the ball which is between them. She moves the ball forwards, backwards and to both sides, and the patient follows the movement with his foot (Fig. 9.35). The patient keeps his trunk vertical and his supporting hip stationary, only his sound leg allowing the movement of the ball.

The patient stands on his sound leg and places his hemiplegic foot on the ball. The therapist may need to help him to bring the foot into a relaxed position without the toes flexing.

Once again she moves the ball in different directions and the patient follows its movement with his hemiplegic leg. He tries to let the movement take place without resistance and with his foot so relaxed that it can contour to the ball's surface (Fig. 9.36a, b). Care must be taken that the patient is not making

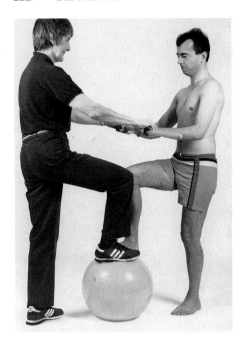

Fig. 9.35. Standing on the hemiplegic leg with the other foot on a ball (left hemiplegia)

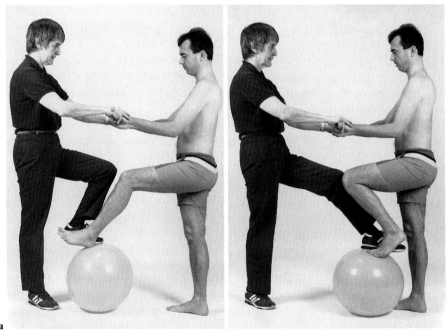

a   b

Fig. 9.36 a, b. Following the movement of the ball with the hemiplegic leg (left hemiplegia)

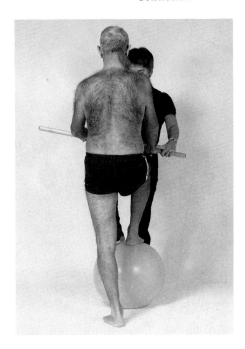

Fig. 9.37. Making a compensatory movement by adducting the hip and shifting
the pelvis laterally (right hemiplegia)

a compensatory movement with his sound hip adducting and his pelvis shifting
laterally to that side (Fig. 9.37).

Regardless of which foot the patient has placed on the ball, the therapist
continues to hold his hemiplegic hand on the pole and is ready at any time to
grasp the pole with her other hand to save the patient should he lose his balance. If the situation becomes precarious, she immediately brings her foot
down to the ground and stabilises the pole firmly so that the patient can use it
to support himself until he is standing with both feet on the floor once more.

9.5 Conclusion

As long as the activity selected is not too difficult for him, the patient will enjoy
working with the ball. Certain of the activities can be included in his home programme as the ball will provide him with control feedback which informs him
whether he is performing the movement correctly. Relatives or friends helping
the more disabled patient to exercise at home will also find it easier to know if
the movement is correct or not by observing the ball and understanding what it
should be doing. Even the simple action of sitting upright on the ball and keeping it stationary stimulates co-ordinated activity in the muscles of the trunk.
The patient can be advised to sit in this way for certain periods each day, perhaps while he watches a favourite television programme or talks to his grand-
children.

10 Walking

Walking is one of the most universal of all human activities (Murray et al. 1964) and the word "walk", in all its forms, has been used not only in poetry, but also in association with many other aspects of our lives, both functional and cultural. Walking enhances and enriches our daily life, broadens our possibilities for achievement and enjoyment, and lightens our work load. It means far more to us than the textbook explanation of locomotion being "the translation of the centre of gravity through space along a path requiring the least expenditure of energy (Basmajian 1979), or the classic dictionary definitions:

- Walking: "The action of moving on the feet at any pace short of breaking into a run or trot".
- Walk: "Of human beings or other bipeds: to progress by alternate movements of the legs so that one foot is always on the ground".

The Shorter Oxford Dictionary (1985) presents, in addition, many other uses such as:

- To go from place to place; to journey, wander.
- To go about in public, live, move (in a place or region).
- To move about or go from place to place on foot for the sake of exercise, pleasure or pastime
- To walk (out) with, said of a young man and young woman keeping company with a view to marriage
- To conduct oneself, behave (ill or well etc.) after Bible examples. To walk with God interpreted to mean 'to lead a godly life' or to have intimate communication with God.

Combined as in 'walk of life' the word refers to social status, rank, trade, profession or occupation.

Walk is given as being the distinctive manner of walking of an individual. "By her graceful walk, the Queen of Love is known" (Dryden, quoted in Shorter Oxford Dictionary 1985).

It is clear, then, that walking with all its associations has a special significance for human beings, and its re-education therefore plays a most important role in rehabilitation. Certainly every patient with hemiplegia longs to be able to walk again, with all that it implies for him. Learning to walk is a goal which he can understand and picture, an aim which has meaning for him.

The ability to walk without a cane or crutch has many advantages. The patient will be able to use his sound hand to carry out tasks as it will not be occupied with holding on for support. If the patient is to walk functionally and for pleasure, his walking must be safe, automatic and not require too great an expenditure of energy. He cannot be expected to walk in such a way, though, until he has achieved sufficient control of his lower limb and trunk by practising the activities described in the previous chapters and in *Steps to Follow* (Davies 1985).

10.1 Observing, Analysing and Facilitating Walking – Theoretical Considerations

Many authors have presented different aspects of normal walking or locomotion, and some have analysed the difficulties experienced by patients with hemiplegia as well. Reading their contributions will help the therapist to understand the problems and enable her to treat the patient more effectively (Basmajian 1979; Brooks 1986; Davies 1985; Klein-Vogelbach 1986; Knuttson 1981; Montgomery 1987; Murray et al. 1964; Perry 1969; Saunders et al. 1953). Some fundamental elements of walking and the parts of the body involved should be considered when observing or facilitating walking.

10.1.1 Rhythm and Cadence

Normal gait is rhythmic and almost effortless, and most people walk between 0.91 and 1.52 m/s or between 112 and 120 steps per min. The duration of each cycle, i. e. the time interval between successive heel strikes of the same foot, is approximately 1 s. At this speed "energy consumption" is minimized, and yet a reasonable propulsion speed is possible. Basmajian (1979) writes: "when a subject is permitted to walk without the imposition of a pace frequency constraint, he selects a walking pace for the set speed in such a manner as to allow a minimum of muscular activity".

The rhythmic nature of walking is easy to recognise because both feet meet the floor with the same amount of force and produce the same sound as they do so. Even when turning around the rhythm remains, one step following another.

10.1.2 Step Length

The step taken with the right foot is the same length as that taken with the left, the mean step length being about 78 cm long. Older people tend to show a decrease in step length, and taller people usually have a greater step length than shorter subjects. The stance phase is the same for both legs, equivalent to about

60% of the walking cycle, and the swinging left leg travels through the air at the same speed as the right one does, taking about 40% of the complete cycle. For a short period, approximately ⅟₁₀ of a second, both feet are in contact with the floor, the double-limb support phase.

10.1.3 Position of the Feet on the Floor

The foot which is swinging forwards to make a step reaches the floor in front with the heel first, the ankle dorsiflexed. At the end of the stance phase the great toe leaves the ground last as the swing phase begins.

When they reach the floor in front, the feet have a similar position in relation to the plane of progression. The angle which is formed between the long axis of each foot and the plane is approximately equal; it is caused by the amount of rotation at the hip and pelvis.

The distance between the feet, or stride width, is less than the distance between the two hip joints. In the study presented by Murray et al. (1964) the mean stride width was 0.8 cm. Klein-Vogelbach (1987) postulates that the swinging foot leaves just enough clearance to avoid its movement being impeded by touching the contralateral leg as the step is made. The relatively narrow base is important because if the limbs were parallel there would need to be excessive and uneconomical lateral displacement of the centre of gravity to transfer the weight over each supporting leg (Saunders et al. 1953).

10.1.4 The Knee

The knee is never fully extended during the stance phase, nor is it held in an excessive amount of flexion. As the body moves forward over the standing leg the knee extends, but remains about 5°–10° short of the amount of extension assumed in a standing posture. When the whole cycle is considered, the knee is at its straightest just before heel strike during the swing phase as the leg extends to attain the required step length.

At the end of the stance phase, the knee flexes rapidly for the initiation of the swing phase, preceding the flexion of the hip, and flexes further as it shortens the leg in the mid-swing position. The knee flexion conserves energy by the shortening of the pendulum as the leg swings forwards with adequate clearance.

The hip joints move forwards continuously throughout the walking cycle, and never backwards. There is no obvious abduction or adduction, despite the muscle activity required. The hip flexes to only about 30° during the swing phase, and as the name implies the movement of the leg is more reactive, resulting from the forward momentum of the body rather than an active lifting of the leg. Once the hip flexion excursion is completed, at about 85% of the cycle, the hip remains in that relative position until the cycle ends at heel strike. At the end of the stance phase the hip extends about 10° more than it does in a standing posture.

10.1.5 The Pelvis

During walking the pelvis remains relatively level, tipping anteriorly and posteriorly through only about 3°. It also tips laterally, so that the side of the swinging leg is a few degrees lower than that of the weight-bearing limb. Some pelvic rotation occurs, closely related to the position of the limbs, the pelvis advancing on the side of the leg swinging forward. Interestingly, Murray et al. (1964) write that: "The absence of pelvic rotation in some of our normal subjects suggests that this is not an obligatory element of normal gait, but rather a convenient excursion, available when walking and, perhaps, attitude demand it."

10.1.6 The Trunk

The trunk is erect and "as the extremities move in an orderly sequence, the trunk is translated forward." (Murray et al. 1964). The forward motion in the plane of progression is almost constant, but there are slight waves of increased and decreased rates of displacement, which are usually imperceptible to the observer. The thorax remains in an upright position without any lateral flexion of the trunk occurring, so that the shoulders stay level with one another.

There is less thoracic rotation than pelvic rotation, and in the opposite direction, so that the right side of the thorax moves forwards with the left side of the pelvis and vice versa. The rotation takes place mainly in the lower thoracic and lumbar spine.

When the walking speed is reduced to less than 70 steps per min, rotation ceases (Klein-Vogelbach 1987).

10.1.7 The Arms

The arms swing back and forth alternately at a normal walking speed, with respect to trunk rotation. The right arm advances with the left leg and vice versa. When the walking speed has been sufficiently reduced, the arms no longer swing as thoracic rotation stops.

It is not essential for the arms to swing. During functional activities arm movement can be voluntarily inhibited in order to carry a tray or other objects steadily.

10.1.8 The Head

During walking the head is not necessarily held in a fixed position, but can be turned or tilted without changing the walking pattern. The eyes are therefore free to look around, at the ground, at the sky or in either direction to the side. When the direction of walking is changed the head usually rotates automatically in that direction, as if initiating the movement.

10.1.9 Maintaining Balance

The ability to take quick automatic steps in any direction enables us to regain our balance should we stumble, trip, or move to avoid other people or objects in our path. Should the surface beneath our feet move, for example in an aeroplane or train, we maintain our balance in the same way. When walking on uneven ground, adjusting steps in the appropriate direction prevent us from losing our balance. Subtle postural adjustments throughout the body take place during free walking to allow for various displacements of the body's centre of gravity without losing balance.

10.2 Facilitating Walking – Practical Considerations

Before walking can be facilitated it is essential that the patient has sufficient active extension in his affected lower limb. If he is encouraged to walk before he is able to take weight on his leg, albeit with help, then he will be forced to use a compensatory movement. He will either push his hip backwards to straighten his knee mechanically or plantarflex the ankle strongly to achieve knee extension. Both of these patterns will result in hyperextension of the knee, with the knee extensors inactive. A self-reinforcing situation results; the patient will learn only to lock his knee, and extensor spasticity will increase, particularly in the plantar flexors of the ankle and foot. "If unchecked, improper motor control can become a highly reinforced program" (Bach-y-Rita and Balliet 1987), and it will be difficult for the patient to change the pattern later. The preparation of the stance phase is a prerequisite for walking, and the activities in lying, sitting and standing positions must be carefully practised.

10.2.1 Footwear

The individual components of gait are practised with the patient barefooted so that activity can be directly stimulated and observed. If the patient cannot dorsiflex his foot selectively, however, then he should wear shoes when walking is facilitated. The sole of the shoe will prevent his toes from being scraped against the floor should they flex during the swing phase, and he will be able to walk more freely as a result. Without shoes the patient will otherwise lift his hemiplegic leg too actively and bring it carefully forwards when taking a step. The conscious flexing and placing of the leg preclude the rhythmic and automatic nature of walking.

Shoes such as those shown in Figs. 10.16 and 10.34 are recommended for the patient who still has difficulty in controlling his foot when walking.

- The upper of the shoe supports the foot well, fastened firmly with shoelaces, a buckle or a velcro fastener.

- A leather sole allows the foot to swing forwards without its catching on the floor.
- A heel of sufficient height brings the patient's weight forward and acts as a substitute for inadequate push off.
- The heel is covered with a nonslip material.
- Both the heel and the sole of the shoe are relatively broad to provide a stable base.

10.2.2 Assisting Hip Extension

Until the patient is able to take weight on his hemiplegic leg without the knee hyperextending, the therapist will need to place her hands directly on his pelvis and use them as an accessory hip extensor, thus preventing the hip joint from moving backwards. She places her thumb over the area of the head of the femur and guides it forwards over the patient's foot (Fig. 10.1a, b). Her other hand rests on the opposite side of his pelvis. Her arm against the patient's thorax gives him added confidence and can help to take some of his weight if necessary.

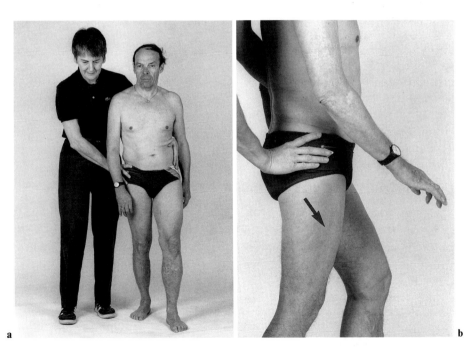

Fig. 10.1 a, b. Keeping the hip forward during the stance and swing phase of walking (right hemiplegia). **a** The therapist walks beside the patient. One of her hands prevents any backward movement of the hip, the other helps with weight transference. **b** The therapist's thumb placed over the head of the femur assists hip extension and prevents hyperextension of the knee

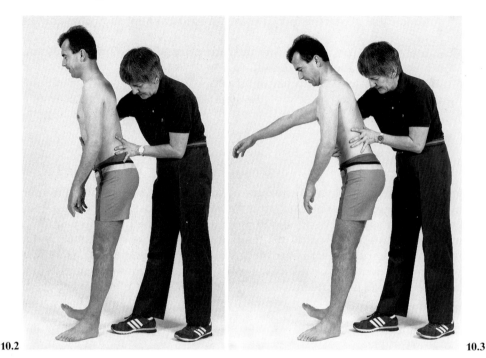

10.2   10.3

Fig. 10.2. Teaching the patient how to react when his weight is drawn backwards (left hemiplegia)

Fig. 10.3. Facilitating balance reactions when the patient's weight is shifted unexpectedly backwards (left hemiplegia)

10.3 Facilitating Walking Backwards

For the patient to feel confident and be safe when walking or standing, he must be able to regain his balance when falling backwards. He will also need to move backwards actively, in order to align his position before sitting down or to move himself out of the way of other people or objects. Learning to walk backwards correctly will also improve the movement components required for walking forwards.

10.3.1 Tipped Backwards Without Taking a Step

The therapist stands behind the patient, one of her hands over his abdomen and the other against his lumbar spine. She draws his weight backwards and uses her hands to move his trunk forwards, in a normal reaction pattern (Fig. 10.2). The patient otherwise tends to hold his body fully extended and would fall over backwards.

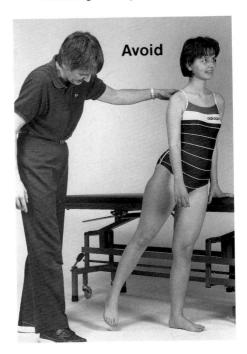

Fig. 10.4. Taking a step backwards using the total pattern of extension (right hemiplegia)

The weight displacement is carried out slowly at first, and within a small range, with the patient consciously performing the correct movements. The therapist shifts the patient's weight progressively further backwards and also increases the speed of the movement (Fig. 10.3). Finally, she should be able to bring him out of balance without warning and the reaction occur automatically.

10.3.2 Taking Steps Backwards

When asked to take a step backwards, the untrained patient will invariably do so by elevating the side of his pelvis and moving his leg back in the total pattern of extension, using his back extensors (Fig. 10.4).

The therapist kneels at the side of the patient and moves his leg in the correct pattern. With one of her hands she holds his toes in dorsal extension and with her other hand over his buttock helps him to prevent hitching his pelvis upwards and backwards as the leg moves (Fig. 10.5a). The patient stands at first with a plinth or table at his sound side, so that he can support himself with his hand as required. The therapist instructs the patient not to resist the movement of his leg and to feel how it should be performed. If he tries to move actively, the extension at the hip may evoke extension at the knee and ankle as well. Moving the foot back in small steps with the knee flexing avoids sudden

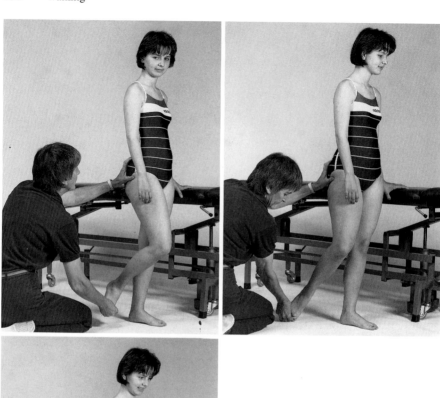

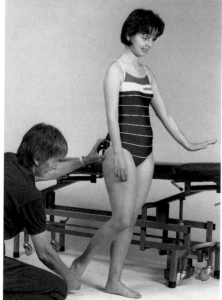

Fig. 10.5 a–c. Learning to take steps backwards (right hemiplegia). **a** Feeling the correct movement as the therapist moves the leg. **b** Letting the foot remain in a relaxed position without pushing against the floor. **c** Taking a normal step backwards without the support of the sound hand

total extension. When the therapist feels that she can move the leg back without it being resisted and without the side of the pelvis moving simultaneously, she asks the patient to take the small steps with her, and he helps actively. Gradually she reduces the amount of assistance she is giving.

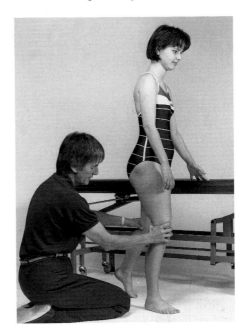

Fig. 10.6. Giving the sound leg a rest. With all the weight taken by the hemiplegic leg, the sound knee flexes and extends rhythmically (right hemiplegia)

When his foot is behind him, the patient leaves it resting there without pushing against the floor. The therapist tells him to let his heel fall inwards towards the other leg to avoid the plantar inversion component of the spastic pattern of extension (Fig. 10.5 b).

As he learns to carry out the movements, the patient tries to repeat them without supporting himself with his sound hand on the plinth (Fig. 10.5 c).

The activity required for standing on the sound leg is tiring, and the therapist needs to alternate the movement with weight moving over the hemiplegic leg as well. Leaving his sound leg behind him, the patient flexes and extends the knee, with no movement occurring in the affected leg (Fig. 10.6).

When the patient can take a step backwards with the hemiplegic foot, the therapist helps him to lower the heel to the ground as he takes a step backwards with his sound leg. With her other hand she also assists the patient in keeping his knee forwards (Fig. 10.7 a, b).

When the movement components have been practised, and the patient has taken over actively with only slight help, the therapist stands behind him and facilitates walking backwards.

With one hand over his abdomen to assist the forward inclination of the trunk and the other behind his pelvis on the hemiplegic side to keep it level, the therapist draws the patient's weight backwards and asks him to take some steps (Fig. 10.8 a, b).

The speed of walking backwards is progressively increased until the therapist can move the patient backwards rather suddenly, and the steps occur spontaneously and quickly.

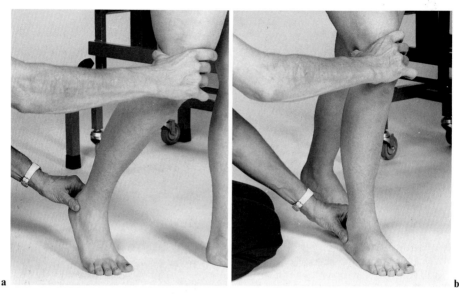

Fig. 10.7 a, b. Taking steps backward (right hemiplegia). **a** When the hemiplegic foot is behind, the therapist helps the patient to lower her heel to the floor without extending her knee. **b** The patient takes a step back with her sound leg and places the foot on the floor parallel to her other foot

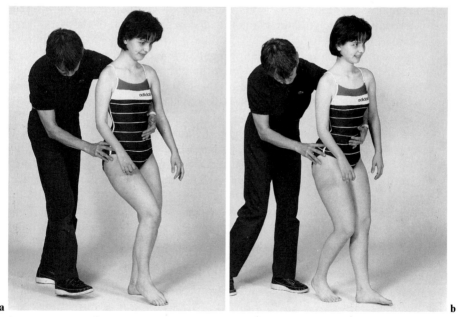

Fig. 10.8 a, b. Facilitating walking backwards (right hemiplegia). **a** The therapist prevents the pelvis from moving backwards. **b** She keeps the patient's trunk forwards as the heel sinks to the floor

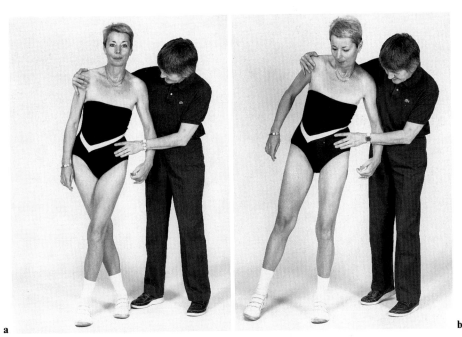

a   b

Fig. 10.9 a, b. Learning to walk sideways towards the sound side (left hemiplegia). **a** The therapist helps the patient to place her hemiplegic foot flat on the floor. **b** She supports the patient when the sound leg leaves the floor

10.4 Facilitating Walking Sideways

In order to walk safely without losing his balance the patient must be able to take quick repeated steps to either side, one foot crossing over in front of the other. He will also need to step to the side to avoid other people coming towards him or objects which are in his way. The muscle activity required for walking sideways can also help to improve his gait pattern.

10.4.1 Towards the Sound Side

The therapist stands beside the patient and places one hand over his pelvis on the hemiplegic side and her other on his sound shoulder. The patient takes a step towards the sound side, crossing his hemiplegic leg over in front of the other one. He tries to place the foot in line with and parallel to the sound foot. He then takes a step with the sound leg and continues to walk sideways in this way (Fig. 10.9 a, b).

Alternatively the therapist can place her hand on the patient's pelvis on the sound side and use her arm against his thorax to lengthen the over-active un-

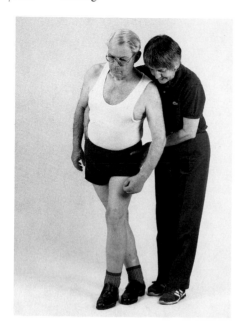

Fig. 10.10. Facilitating walking towards the sound side. The therapist uses her arm to allow the trunk to lengthen on the overactive sound side

affected side of his trunk as he moves his hemiplegic leg in front of the other (Fig. 10.10).

10.4.2 Towards the Hemiplegic Side

The therapist stands next to the patient on the affected side. With one hand in his axilla she lengthens the side of his trunk and with the other on the opposite side of his pelvis she shifts his weight laterally over the hemiplegic leg. The patient brings his sound leg sideways crossing it over in front of the other. He aims at placing the feet parallel to, and in line with one another as he continues walking sideways (Fig. 10.11 a–c). The patient prevents his knee from hyper-extending, which is only possible if he moves his pelvis sufficiently far over the hemiplegic leg.

Many patients will have difficulty in bringing the hemiplegic leg out from behind the other leg in order to take the next step sideways as the movement requires considerable selection, i. e. knee flexion while the hip is extended. The therapist facilitates the movement by allowing a backward rotation of the side of the trunk and pelvis at first, which she gradually eliminates as control improves.

When the patient can control the movements of his pelvis and legs, the therapist places her hands on his shoulders and moves him sideways as he takes repeated steps, first to one side and then to the other (Fig. 10.12 a, b). The activity is performed slowly and carefully at first.

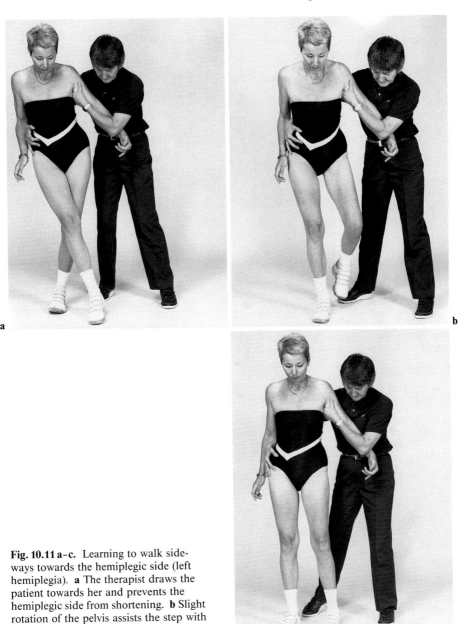

Fig. 10.11 a–c. Learning to walk sideways towards the hemiplegic side (left hemiplegia). **a** The therapist draws the patient towards her and prevents the hemiplegic side from shortening. **b** Slight rotation of the pelvis assists the step with the affected leg. **c** The patient steps to the side with the hemiplegic foot

As the patient's ability and confidence improve, the therapist decreases her support and increases the speed of the movement sideways. She holds his hemiplegic arm lightly, and he follows the unexpected and rapid direction changes without hesitation (Fig. 10.13 a, b).

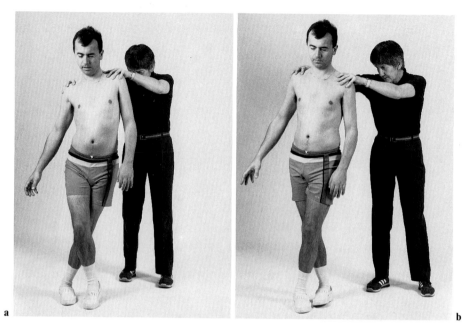

Fig. 10.12 a, b. Walking sideways with facilitation from the shoulders (left hemiplegia) **a** towards the hemiplegic side and **b** towards the sound side

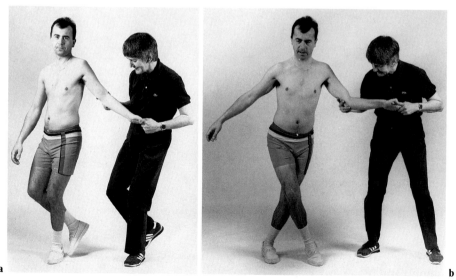

Fig. 10.13 a, b. Taking quick steps to either side with unexpected changes in direction (left hemiplegia) **a** to the sound side and **b** to the hemiplegic side

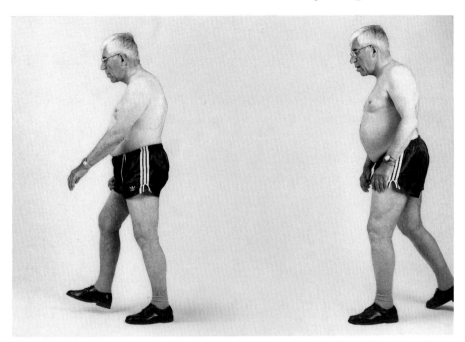

Fig. 10.14. When the centre of gravity is too far back, the swing phase is active instead of reactive (right hemiplegia)

10.5 Facilitating Walking Forwards

10.5.1 Stabilising the Thorax and Moving the Trunk Forwards

Many patients will be unable to maintain extension of the thoracic spine or prevent side flexion of the trunk when they walk. They will also keep their centre of gravity too far back, which prevents a normal, reactive swing phase from occurring. Instead the leg is lifted actively to take a step (Fig. 10.14).

The therapist walks beside the patient and stabilises his thorax in extension. She places one hand in front of his rib cage at about the level of the end of his sternum and her other hand posteriorly at approximately the same level, with the thumbs uppermost (Fig. 10.15). Holding the thorax firmly between her hands in the correct position, she translates it forwards along the plane of walking, and the patient moves his legs accordingly. The therapist can also take some of the weight of the patient's trunk as he moves (Fig. 10.16).

When the speed of the walking is appropriate, she can introduce some rotation of the trunk with her hands.

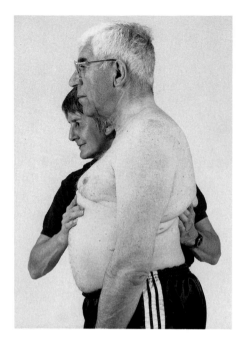

Fig. 10.15. Stabilising the thoracic spine and supporting some of the patient's weight (right hemiplegia)

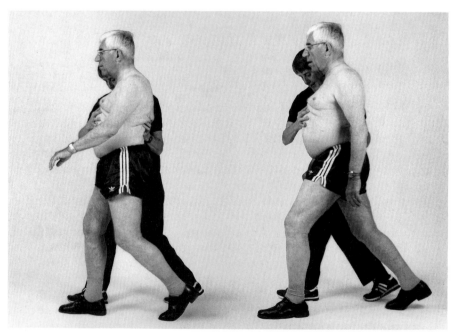

Fig. 10.16. Facilitating the reactive swing phase with increase of step length (compare with Fig. 10.14; right hemiplegia)

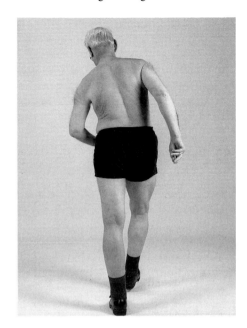

Fig. 10.17. Difficulty in keeping the shoulders level and an associated reaction of the arm in flexion (left hemiplegia)

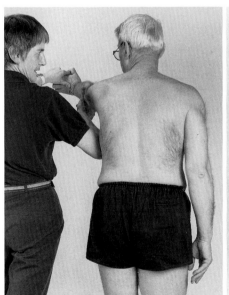

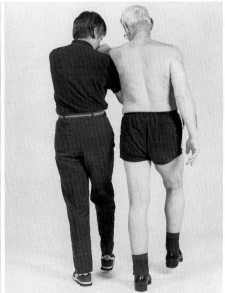

a   b

Fig. 10.18 a, b. Facilitating walking with the arm held forwards and extended (posterior view; left hemiplegia). **a** The therapist inhibits depression of the shoulder girdle and spastic flexion of the arm and hand. **b** She brings the centre of gravity forwards and keeps the ribs down with her upper arm

10.5.2 Facilitation to Prevent Side Flexion of the Trunk and Associated Reactions in the Arm

The patient may have difficulty in keeping his shoulders level, and the depression of the hemiplegic shoulder may be combined with an associated reaction of the arm which pulls into the spastic pattern of flexion (Fig. 10.17). The shoulder may, however, be equally depressed even though the arm appears to be hypotonic.

10.5.2.1 Supporting the Hemiplegic Arm

The therapist walks beside the patient, holding his extended hemiplegic arm forwards with about 90° flexion of the shoulder. With the hand nearest to the patient she supports the elbow in extension and lifts the shoulder to its correct level. Her hand is just proximal to the humeral condyles and with her upper arm against the patient's ribs she applies counter-pressure to correct the position of his thorax, i. e. she abducts her arm and moves the patient's ribs down and away from her. Her other hand keeps the patient's wrist and fingers extended, her index finger maintaining his thumb in an abducted extended position (Fig. 10.18 a, b).

Using her thumb on the dorsum of his hand and her other hand over his humeral condyles, the therapist draws the patient's weight forwards as they walk rhythmically together (Fig. 10.19 a, b).

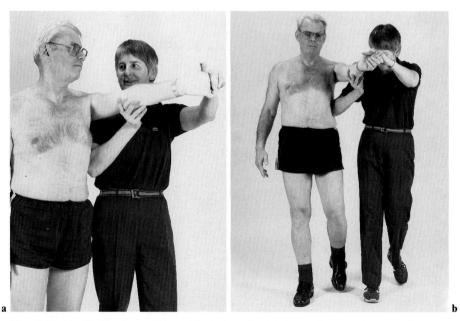

Fig. 10.19 a, b. Facilitating walking with the arm held forwards in extension (anterior view; left hemiplegia). **a** Starting position. **b** Walking

10.5.2.2 Holding a Ball

Holding a large ball in his arms will also help the patient to bring his centre of gravity further forwards, take longer steps and prevent associated reactions in the arm. Standing in front of the patient and facing him, the therapist helps him to encircle the gymnastic ball with both his arms, his hands lying flat on it and his shoulders level. Walking backwards, but rhythmically the therapist draws the patient gently forwards (Fig. 10.20a–c). Once the appropriate cadence of

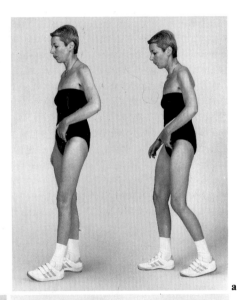

Fig. 10.20 a–c. Facilitating walking with a gymnastic ball held in both arms (left hemiplegia). **a** Difficulty in stabilising the thoracic spine, small careful steps and increased flexor spasticity in the arm. **b** The therapist holds the patient's hand lightly on the ball and draws the weight forwards. **c** Free flowing steps of normal length

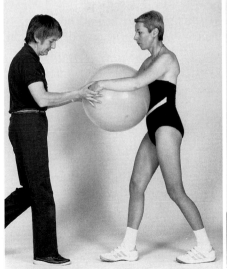

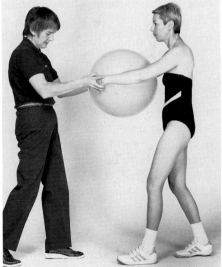

walking has been reached the therapist can introduce trunk rotation by moving the ball slightly from one side to the other.

10.5.2.3 Holding a Pole in Both Hands

If the patient moves his trunk backwards to bring his hemiplegic foot forwards by extending the sound hip, the step will be too short and the arm will tend to pull into flexion (Fig. 10.21). The therapist places a rounded wooden pole in the patient's hemiplegic hand and, making sure that the wrist is dorsiflexed, places the pole against her chest (Fig. 10.22a). The pole against her body keeps the patient's fingers in a grasping position. With one hand beneath the hemiplegic arm the therapist keeps the patient's elbow extended and the pole against her, at the same time keeping his shoulder in line from below. The patient then grasps the pole with his other hand, so that his arms are parallel and his hands shoulder width apart. Holding the sound arm with her other hand the therapist ensures that both shoulders are level with one another (Fig. 10.22b).

She asks the patient to lean forward on the pole against her chest, taking care that he does not do so by extending his lumbar spine and pushing his navel towards her (Fig. 10.22c). The axis of movement should be only through his ankle joints.

The therapist enables the patient to achieve exactly the right amount of forward inclination by indicating to him how much pressure she is feeling. For example, should he be pushing too energetically, she asks him to reduce the weight by "2 kg" (Fig. 10.23a). Once the starting position has been adjusted the patient walks forward, maintaining the pressure of the pole at a constant against the therapist's chest (Fig. 10.23b, c). If the pressure does not vary, the hip is not moving backwards at any time during the walking cycle. Both the swing phase and stance phase are automatically improved, and the step lengths become more normal. The patient's weight is no longer behind his centre of gravity, and he does not have to move his trunk backwards in order to lift his hemiplegic leg forwards.

10.5.2.4 Applying Pressure to the Patient's Chest

Patients who have difficulty in bringing their hemiplegic leg forwards in the swing phase resort to using many different compensatory movements to make the step. Many will use extension of their sound hip to rock the trunk backwards in order to bring the hemiplegic leg forwards or will hitch up the pelvis on that side. Some will go up on the toes of the sound foot to provide more clearance for the hemiplegic foot even when wearing a dorsal flexion-assisting brace or calliper (Fig. 10.24).

The therapist places the dorsal aspect of her relaxed fingers against the lower third of the patient's sternum, with flexion of her metacarpalphalangeal joints. Holding her wrist in a neutral position and her elbow extended, she asks the patient to lean his weight against her hand, keeping his trunk in a straight

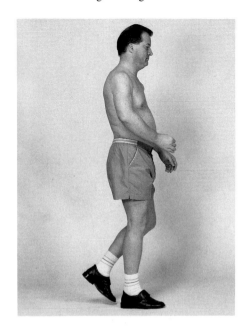

Fig. 10.21. The patient's trunk is inclined backwards during the stance and swing phase. The step length is reduced and the arm pulls into flexion (right hemiplegia)

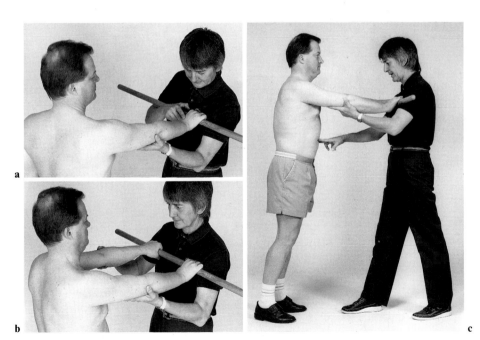

Fig. 10.22 a–c. Facilitating walking with a pole held in both hands, adjusting the starting position (right hemiplegia). **a** The hemiplegic hand is brought into place with the wrist in extension. **b** Both hands on the pole with the shoulders level and elbows straight. **c** Leaning forward from the ankles

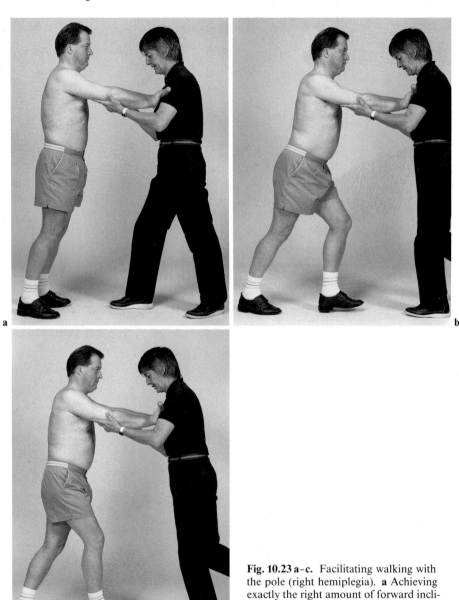

Fig. 10.23 a–c. Facilitating walking with the pole (right hemiplegia). **a** Achieving exactly the right amount of forward inclination. **b** The pressure of the pole against the therapist remains constant. **c** The hemiplegic leg swings forward

line. The fulcrum of the forward movement is only in his ankle joints (Fig. 10.25 a).

Because his weight is forward and his abdominal muscles active, the hemiplegic leg will often swing forward with far less effort, and he will no longer

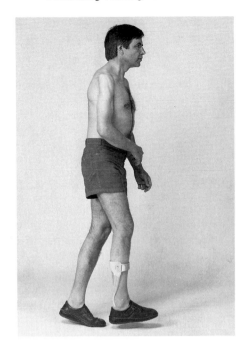

Fig. 10.24. Pushing up on the toes of the sound foot to bring the hemiplegic leg forwards, despite a foot brace (right hemiplegia)

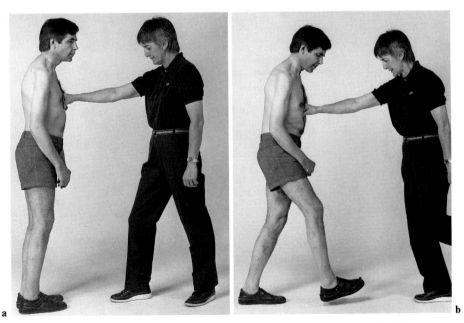

Fig. 10.25 a, b. Facilitating walking with pressure applied against the lower end of the sternum (right hemiplegia). **a** The patient leans forwards from the ankles, his weight supported by the therapist's extended arm. **b** The hemiplegic foot clears the ground easily, without the ankle support

need to lean backwards, hitch up his pelvis or go up on the toes of his sound leg (Fig. 10.25 b).

10.5.3 Facilitation Using Stimulating and Inhibitory Tapping

Both pressure tapping to increase activity in a muscle group and inhibitory tapping to inhibit an abnormal movement pattern can be used in the facilitation of walking. Exact timing of the tapping is crucial.

10.5.3.1 Stimulating Tapping over the Hip Extensors

Hip extension can be stimulated by tapping firmly over the muscle group at the very onset of the stance phase, i. e. at the moment of heel strike or when the patient's foot meets the floor and his hip would otherwise move backwards as the leg accepts his weight (Fig. 10.26a).

Walking at his side and slightly in front of him, the therapist holds the patient's hemiplegic arm forwards, using the hand furthest from him to support beneath his elbow. She draws the patient's weight forward, with his arm held at a right angle to his trunk.

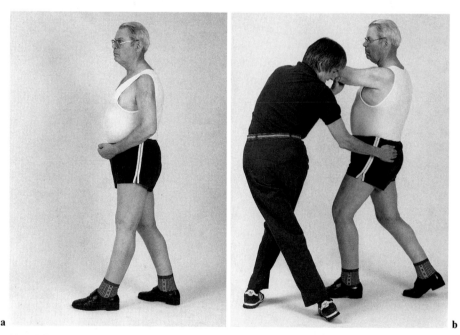

a   b

Fig. 10.26 a, b. Stimulating tapping to correct the stance phase (left hemiplegia). **a** The patient's knee hyperextends at the beginning of the stance phase. **b** The therapist's cupped hand taps firmly downwards and forwards over the hip extensors at heel strike

As the patient walks the therapist uses the cupped palm of her other hand to tap firmly downwards and forwards over his buttock on the hemiplegic side, just as his foot reaches the floor (Fig. 10.26b). She keeps her hand in firm contact until the hemiplegic leg starts its movement forwards. During the swing

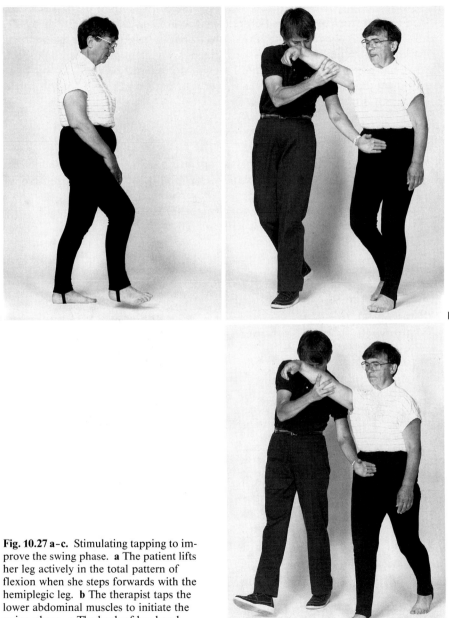

Fig. 10.27 a–c. Stimulating tapping to improve the swing phase. a The patient lifts her leg actively in the total pattern of flexion when she steps forwards with the hemiplegic leg. b The therapist taps the lower abdominal muscles to initiate the swing phase. c The back of her hand maintains contact until heel strike

phase she moves her arm well back preparatory to bringing her hand down firmly on to the hip extensors at the beginning of the next stance phase.

10.5.3.2 Stimulating Tapping for the Lower Abdominal Muscles

The swing phase can be initiated and facilitated by holding the patient's extended arm in front of him, as before. The therapist uses the back of her other hand to tap briskly over the patient's lower abdominals at the precise moment when knee flexion to initiate the swing phase of the hemiplegic leg begins. She lets her hand remain in contact until weight acceptance on the leg. Her hand moves away during the stance phase, ready to perform the tap for the subsequent swing (Fig. 10.27 a–c).

10.5.3.3 Inhibitory Tapping

If the patient tends to hitch his pelvis up and back at the beginning of the swing phase (Fig. 10.28 a), the therapist can inhibit the abnormal pattern by using inhibitory tapping.

She helps the patient to transfer his weight forwards as he walks by holding his hemiplegic arm in front of him with the elbow extended.

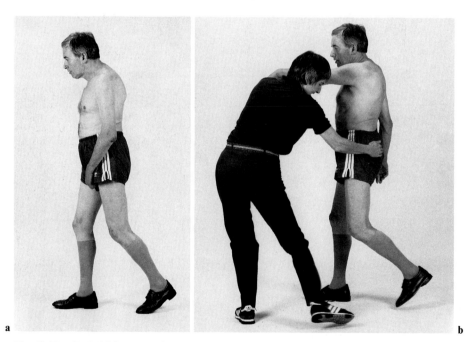

a   b

Fig. 10.28 a, b. Inhibitory tapping to correct the initiation of the swing phase (left hemiplegia). **a** The patient hitches his pelvis up and back as he prepares to make a step. **b** The therapist's cupped hand taps firmly forwards and downwards over the patient's buttock

With the palm of her other hand the therapist taps firmly forwards and downwards over his buttock to inhibit the backward and upward movement of the pelvis just before it would otherwise occur, i. e. at the very onset of the swing phase (Fig. 10.28 b). Her hand remains in contact with the gluteal region until weight acceptance on that leg, and then she moves it away, ready to tap again for the following step.

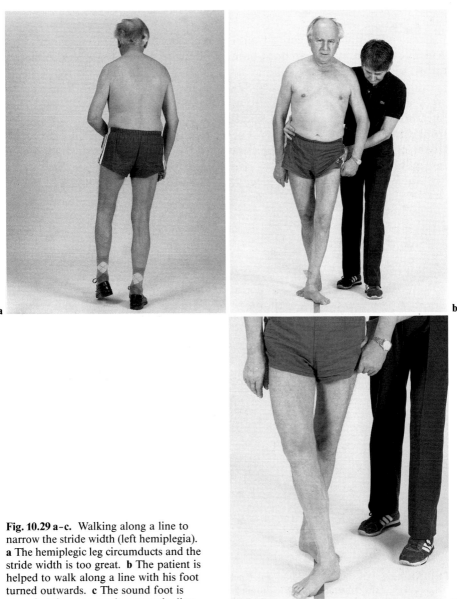

Fig. 10.29 a–c. Walking along a line to narrow the stride width (left hemiplegia). **a** The hemiplegic leg circumducts and the stride width is too great. **b** The patient is helped to walk along a line with his foot turned outwards. **c** The sound foot is placed at the same angle across the line

10.5.4 Facilitation to Narrow the Stride Width

To compensate for inadequate trunk control and maintain their balance most patients will walk with their feet wider apart than normal. The increased stride width requires a greater lateral shift of the pelvis to bring the weight over the supporting leg for the stance phase (Saunders et al. 1953). Too much energy is spent, and the muscles of the trunk are used abnormally (Fig. 10.29 a).

10.5.4.1 Walking Along a Line

A line is marked out on the floor, either with chalk, paint or a strip of adhesive tape. The patient practises walking along the line with his hips laterally rotated and his feet placed so that the line passes beneath the arch of his foot.

The therapist walks beside the patient and facilitates the movement of his hips. With one hand placed so that her thumb is over the head of the femur from behind, she assists hip extension with external rotation on the hemiplegic side. Her other hand rests on the opposite side of his pelvis to steady him and to help him to place the sound leg correctly on the line in front (Fig. 10.29 b, c).

When the patient is able to place his feet accurately on the line as he walks,

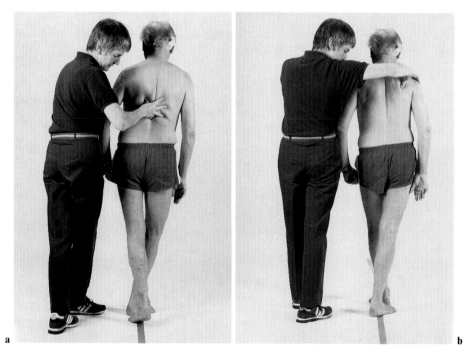

a   b

Fig. 10.30 a, b. Walking along a line with facilitation to stabilise the thoracic spine (left hemiplegia). **a** The therapist supports the thorax from in front and behind. **b** Correcting the position of the shoulders

the therapist can stabilise his thorax by placing one hand over his thoracic spine posteriorly and the other over the sternal angle anteriorly (Fig. 10.30a).

To assist extension of the thoracic spine, the therapist can place her hands on the patient's shoulders, her thumbs over his scapulae. She adducts the scapulae, so helping the patient to overcome the compensatory fixation of the thorax (Fig. 10.30b).

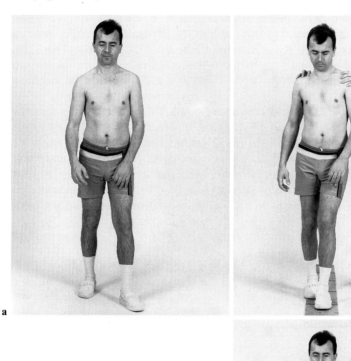

a   b

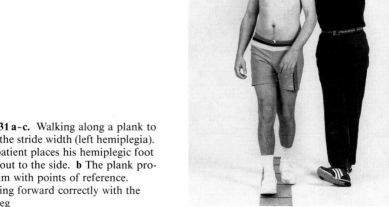

Fig. 10.31 a-c. Walking along a plank to correct the stride width (left hemiplegia). **a** The patient places his hemiplegic foot too far out to the side. **b** The plank provides him with points of reference. **c** Stepping forward correctly with the sound leg

c

10.5.4.2 Walking Along a Plank

When walking alone, the patient will automatically place his feet too far to the side at the end of the swing phase in order to widen his base of support (Fig. 10.31 a). Through repeated use of the wide base it becomes part of his customary walking pattern.

By practising walking along a board on the floor the patient can experience a normal stride width as the board provides points of reference as to where his feet should contact the ground in front of him. Not only does he experience the correct stride width, but selective activity of the trunk is also stimulated. The therapist may need to support his hemiplegic hip at first, but once the legs are moving freely she can reduce her support and give appropriate assistance from his shoulders (Fig. 10.31 b, c).

When he can walk confidently along the plank, the patient holds a gymnastic ball in his arms as he does so. Holding the ball means that he can no longer look at his feet directly, but sees the plank further ahead of him and must feel the position of his feet. Compensatory movements of the sound shoulder and arm are eliminated, and the position of the feet on the plank is attained through the lower trunk and hips (Fig. 10.32 a, b). The therapist helps the patient to keep his hemiplegic arm on the ball without effort if he is still unable to do so himself.

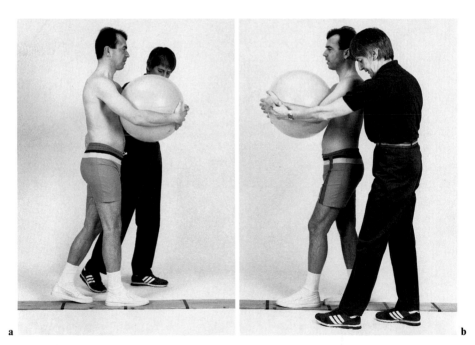

Fig. 10.32 a, b. Walking along the plank without visual control. **a** When holding a ball in his arms, the patient does not look down at his feet. **b** The therapist supports the hemiplegic hand on the ball

10.5.5 Facilitation to Re-establish Rhythm

Patients are often not aware that their walking is not rhythmic or that the rhythm is syncopated. It is helpful to practise activities which provide rhythm while walking. The activities also help to bring weight forwards and to make the walking more automatic, rather than a careful, studied placing of alternate feet in front. There are various reasons for the arhythmic gait pattern, one of the common causes being the hyper-extended knee which causes a delay in bringing the weight over the hemiplegic foot at the beginning of the stance phase (Fig. 10.33 a, b).

10.5.5.1 Using a Tambourine

The patient accompanies his own rhythm with a tambourine, striking it each time his foot reaches the floor in front.

    The therapist helps him to hold the tambourine in front with his hemiplegic hand. Her other hand holds his sound hand on the drumstick and guides it to beat a regular appropriate rhythm striking the tambourine at the exact moment when each foot meets the ground. She can change the tempo, making it slower or faster as required, and the patient moves his legs accordingly to keep time (Fig. 10.34 a).

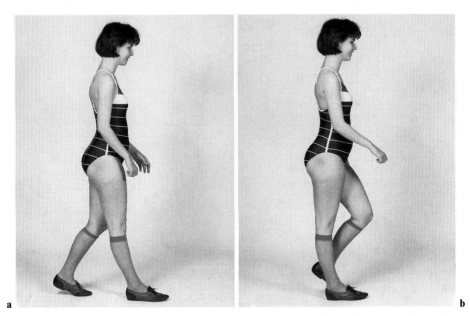

a   b

Fig. 10.33 a, b. Loss of the normal rhythm of gait (right hemiplegia). **a** Hyperextension of the knee at heel strike delays transferring the weight forwards. **b** The hip moves backwards, causing a syncopated rhythm

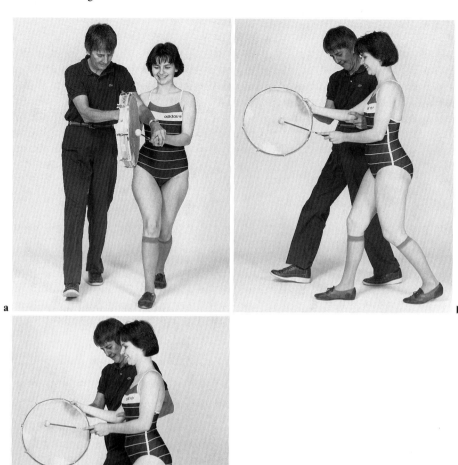

Fig. 10.34 a–c. Using a tambourine to re-establish rhythm (right hemiplegia).
a The therapist holds the patient's hemiplegic hand on the tabourine and guides her sound hand to strike the surface as each foot meets the ground. **b** The patient beats the rhythm herself. **c** Normal step length without hyperextension of the knee

Once the patient is walking rhythmically, the therapist releases his sound hand and he beats the rhythm himself (Fig. 10.34b, c). Should he lose the rhythm after a few steps, she holds his hand again and continues with the correct beat.

The activity can be made progressively more complicated by using two or even three taps on the tambourine for each step, the last tap being simulta-

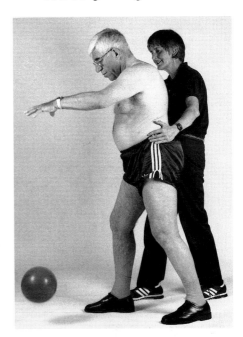

Fig. 10.35. Walking to the rhythm of bouncing and catching a ball with the sound hand (right hemiplegia)

neous with the foot landing on the floor at the end of the swing phase, e. g. ta-ta-*tum,* ta-ta-*tum.*

10.5.5.2 Bouncing a Ball with the Sound Hand

The patient bounces a ball on the floor and then catches it again with his sound hand. He times the bounce so that the ball hits the ground at the same moment as his hemiplegic foot does at the end of the swing phase. His sound leg swings forwards as the ball moves up again, and he catches it as his foot reaches the floor (Fig. 10.35).

The activity not only reinforces rhythm, but also ensures that the sound arm moves forward with the opposite foot, and is not held in a fixed position, e. g. abduction and extension.

10.5.5.3 Bouncing a Large Ball with Both Hands

The patient holds a large ball with both his hands, bouncing it on the floor and catching it again as he walks forwards in a set rhythm. The patient will need to learn to bounce and catch the ball while standing still. The therapist stands beside him and guides both his hands as he picks up the ball, bounces and catches it (Fig. 10.36a–d). If she does not guide his sound hand as well, he will attempt to grasp the ball with it from below.

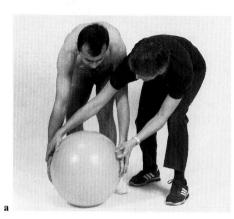

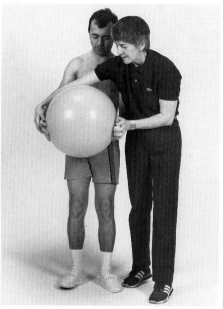

Fig. 10.36 a–d. Learning to bounce and catch a ball with both hands while standing (left hemiplegia). **a** The therapist guides both the patient's hands to pick up the ball from the floor. **b** Checking that the patient is not holding the ball too tightly

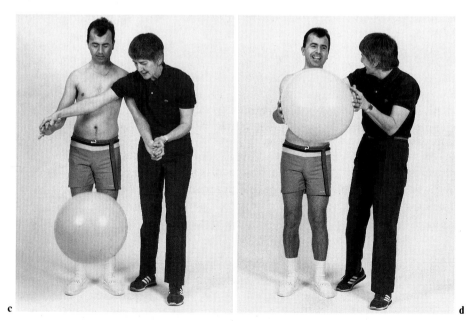

Fig. 10.36. c Bouncing the ball on the floor. **d** Catching the ball in the centre

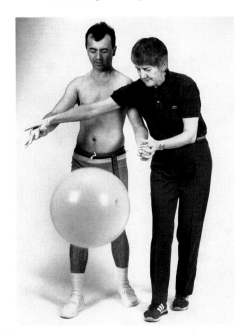

Fig. 10.37. Walking rhythmically, in time
with bouncing and catching the ball.
Both hands are guided by the therapist
(left hemiplegia)

The patient walks forwards, and after taking two steps the therapist bounces the ball with the patient's hands and then catches it again in time with the following two steps, i. e. "step-step-bounce-catch", without interrupting the walking (Fig. 10.37). The ball hits the floor as one of his feet reaches the floor at the end of the swing phase, and he catches the ball at the end of the subsequent swing phase with the opposite foot.

Once the patient can walk in time with the bouncing and catching of the ball, his hands guided by the therapist, she can release his sound hand. First, the patient learns to bounce and catch the ball gently and accurately standing still, with the therapist guiding only his hemiplegic hand appropriately (Fig. 10.38a).

Bouncing and catching is then combined with walking (Fig. 10.38b). If the patient has regained sufficient active movement in his hemiplegic arm, the therapist can gradually reduce the amount of assistance she gives to his affected hand.

10.5.5.4 Imitating the Therapist's Steps

The patient's steps are frequently unequal in length, the sound leg taking a shorter step in the front than the affected one. His arm often has increased flexor tone and pulls into a stiff flexed position due to an associated reaction (Fig. 10.39a).

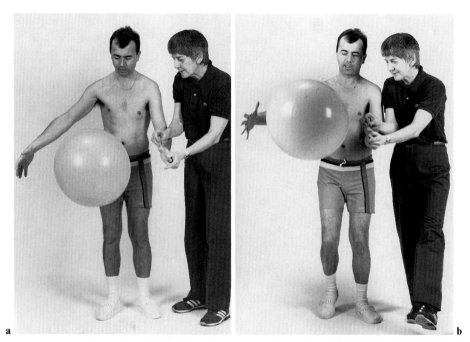

a   b

Fig. 10.38 a, b. Walking in time with bouncing the ball (left hemiplegia). **a** Learning to bounce the ball and catch it, with the therapist guiding only the hemiplegic hand. **b** Walking rhythmically to "step-step bounce-catch".

The therapist walks beside him with his hemiplegic hand clasped in hers. She asks the patient to copy her steps exactly in relation to time and distance, and as they walk she swings his arm freely forwards as he takes a step with his sound leg and backwards as he moves his hemiplegic leg (Fig. 10.39 b).

10.5.6 Facilitating Walking on the Toes

If a more normal gait pattern is to be achieved, then it is essential that the patient be helped to regain active control of plantar flexion of his ankle (Olney et al. 1986; Winter 1983). Many therapists avoid this important aspect of selective activity because they are afraid that spasticity may be increased or clonus elicited. On the contrary, active plantar flexion will inhibit hypertonus in both the plantar flexors of the ankle and the flexors of the toes as long as the movement is performed selectively (see Figs. 8.29, 8.30a, and 8.32a). When the patient is learning to walk on his toes, particular care must be taken that his knee remains forwards over his foot and does not push back into hyperextension in the total pattern of extension. His knee should point directly in the line of his foot and not deviate either medially or laterally. The therapist may need to kneel beside

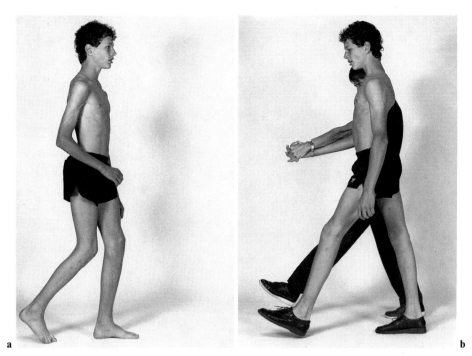

a   b

Fig. 10.39 a, b. Imitating the therapist's steps (right hemiplegia). **a** The patient walks arhythmically, taking a small step with his sound leg with the foot landing flat on the floor. **b** The patient copies the position of the therapist's feet and adopts her rhythm and step length. The therapist clasps the hemiplegic hand and facilitates the arm swing

the patient at first to help him control the position of his knee and also to prevent his toes from flexing as he practises walking on his toes.

Later she can walk beside the patient and facilitate the correct movement by stabilising his thorax and at the same time taking some of his weight (Fig. 10.40). As his control over active plantar flexion improves, the patient can walk with alternating dorsal flexion and plantar flexion of his foot, which is far more difficult for him. At the end of the swing phase, his heel should contact the floor, and, as he takes weight over that foot, he rises up on his toes as the other leg swings forward and the sequence is repeated. He walks with a lilting gait, exaggerating plantar flexion in the stance phase.

10.5.7 Walking with the Head Moving Freely

Most patients tend to walk with their head in a fixed position, usually looking at the ground a short distance in front of them (Fig. 10.41). For walking to be truly functional, the patient must be able to move his head freely without disturbing the rhythm or altering direction.

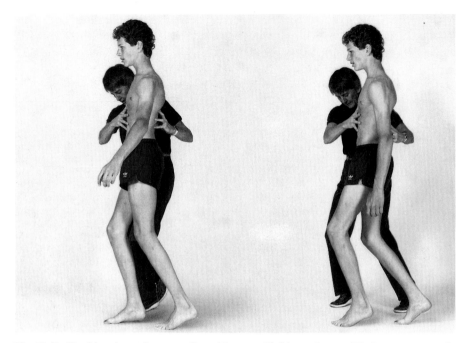

Fig. 10.40. Teaching the patient to walk on his toes with his trunk erect. His knee must remain in a slightly flexed position pointing directly over his foot (right hemiplegia)

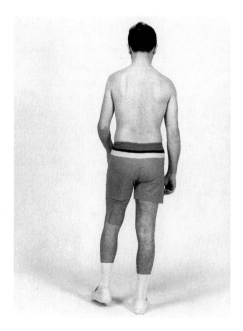

Fig. 10.41. The patient tends to hold his head in a fixed position and look at the ground in front of him (left hemiplegia)

10.5.7.1 Throwing and Catching a Ball

The patient walks forwards and with his sound hand throws a ball to a person walking parallel to him and some distance away. He is asked to look directly into the person's eyes as he does so, and the ball is thrown back for him to catch. The two throw the ball back and forth, and the patient keeps his trunk

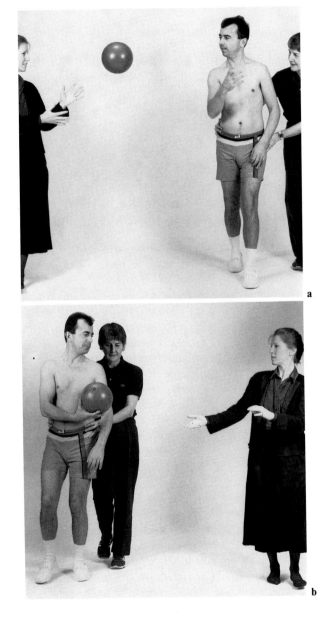

Fig. 10.42 a, b. Walking forwards when the head is turned to one side to throw and catch a ball (left hemiplegia). **a** Looking to the right. **b** Looking to the left

and feet moving forwards in a straight line despite the rotation of his head. The therapist walks next to the patient at his hemiplegic side, but slightly behind to avoid hampering the flight of the ball. Her hands rest lightly on either side of the patient's pelvis, and she gives only as much support as is necessary. The activity is carried out with the helper throwing the ball from the patient's sound side as well as from his hemiplegic side. The walking tempo remains constant (Fig. 10.42a, b).

10.5.7.2 Beating a Tambourine

The patient walks forwards and beats the tambourine which is moved into different positions by the therapist (Fig. 10.43a, b). His walking remains constant with regard to rhythm, speed and direction.

10.6 Conclusion

"Human locomotion is a phenomenon of the most extraordinary complexity" (Saunders et al. 1953). So complex is the motion that attempts to build a computer-controlled machine which can walk have been limited. A construction with six legs imitating an insect-type gait was possible because there was no need for balance reactions. Even a machine which hopped on a single leg could be programmed (Raibert and Sutherland 1983). Apparently the problem of programming two-legged walking with the necessary co-ordination and balance reactions has still to be solved! Normal walking "involves small portions of all joint motions and muscular activity available in the lower extremities, the pelvis and the trunk" (Perry 1969). It is therefore most useful in the limited therapy time available for stimulating activity in many muscles simultaneously. The ability to walk clearly means more than being able to move slowly and laboriously for a number of metres along the smooth floor of the hospital corridor, supported on a cane or crutch.

People walk to enjoy their surroundings, to observe others and interesting things and places, and to talk and share impressions with companions. It may well be that "locomotion does not require control by the cerebral cortex" and that "patterns for locomotion are generated in the spinal cord by central pattern generators (CPGs) that operate in a flexible manner under supraspinal control" (Brooks 1986). Such walking would, however, be without purpose or judgement, and the ability to avoid obstacles in the path or adapt to changing surfaces would be absent. It is important for the patient that he learns to walk on all types of surfaces and up and down hill as well. The activities for facilitating walking should be practised outside as well as indoors, and the patient should experience walking on stones, on grass and on uneven ground.

At first, whether inside or outside, if there is the slightest danger of the patient injuring his ankle due to increased supination of the foot, a supporting bandage can be applied over the shoe, or he can wear a plastic brace to support

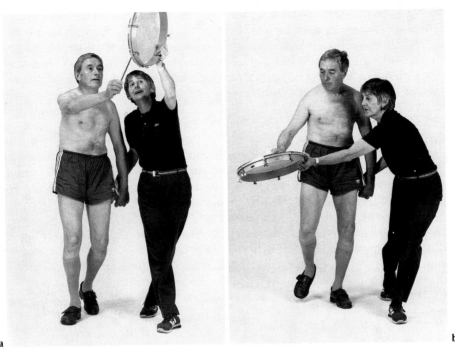

Fig. 10.43 a, b. Moving the head freely without changing the rhythm, speed or direction of walking (left hemiplegia). **a** The therapist holds a tambourine for the patient to beat in time with his steps. **b** She changes the position of the tambourine for each step

his foot while practising the activities described in this chapter. The patient may be able to walk slowly and carefully without his foot being supported. When practising free, flowing walking or bouncing a ball, however, he will not be able to concentrate on placing his foot safely on the ground, nor will the therapist be able to take care of his ankle as she assists him with the various activities. In any event, the aim of the activities is to re-establish automatic walking and it would be counter-productive if the patient needed to be careful and think about the position of his foot all the time. As soon as the patient has regained adequate control over his foot, however, he wears normal everyday shoes and practises walking without the support of a bandage or brace.

The speed of walking needs to be increased to as near normal as possible. If the patient can only walk very slowly, it takes far too long for him to get where he is going and requires far too much energy. Motivation is directly related to that amount of energy required to perform an activity being appropriate for the task. Walking slowly also makes balance far more difficult. The patient's partner or companions find a slow walking pace very frustrating and will frequently go on ahead and then wait for him. As a result he will often have to walk alone, and much of the pleasure of the outing will be lost as he tries desperately to keep up with the other person or persons.

The therapist needs to analyse the patient's walking carefully and practise with him the components which are causing the difficulties. She can then try to use the different ways of facilitating gait as the patient's control improves.

Although the patient may never walk as freely and effortlessly as he did before suffering a hemiplegia, every attempt should be made to achieve safe, automatic walking, with the pattern, rhythm and speed as normal as they possibly can be. Regaining the ability to walk unafraid and unnoticed in the street among others should be the goal of rehabilitation, both for the patient and his therapist. It should always be remembered, however, that during the development of motor skills, the child only accomplishes a normal adult pattern of walking at about 7 years of age (Okamoto 1973). During a period of 6 years it would have repeated 3 million steps to achieve that level of performance, according to Kottke (1978). To expect the patient to re-learn such a highly co-ordinated movement sequence in a few months would be unrealistic. It may even take years before some patients are able to walk freely and confidently again, depending upon the degree of their disability. Others may achieve independent walking in a very short time, but the quality deteriorates if treatment is discontinued too soon. Rehabilitation should, therefore, be regarded as an ongoing process if optimal results are to be attained and then maintained.

It's a long long road,
from which there is no return.
While we're on our way to there
why not share?
And the load
doesn't weigh me down at all.
He ain't heavy
He's my brother.

Neil Diamond

References

Adler MK, Curtland C, Brown JR, Acton P (1980) Stroke rehabilitation – is age a determinant? J Am Geriatr Soc 11: 499–503

Bach-y-Rita P, Balliet R (1987) Recovery from stroke. In: Duncan P, Badke M (eds) Stroke rehabilitation: the recovery of motor control. Year Book Medical, Chicago, pp 81–82

Badke MB, Duncan PW (1983) Patterns of rapid motor responses during postural adjustments when standing in healthy subjects and hemiplegic patients. Phys Ther 63: 13–20

Basmajian JW (1979) Muscles alive. Their functions revealed by electromyography, 4th edn. Williams and Wilkins, Baltimore

Blair MJ (1986) Examination of the thoracic spine. In: Grieve GP (ed) Modern manual therapy of the vertebral column. Churchill Livingstone, Edinburgh

Bobath B (1971) Abnormal postural reflex activity caused by brain lesions. Heinemann, London

Bobath B (1978) Adult hemiplegia: evaluation and treatment, 2nd edn. Heinemann, London

Bobath K (1971) The normal postural reflex mechanism and its deviation in children with cerebral palsy. (Congress lecture, reprint from Physiotherapy, November 1971, pp 1–11)

Bobath K (1980) Neurophysiology, pt 1. Videofilm recorded at the Post-graduate Study Centre, Hermitage, Bad Ragaz

Bobath K, Bobath B (1975) Die Behandlung der Hemiplegie der Erwachsenen. Z Kr Gymn 27: 356–360

Bobath K, Bobath B (1977) Lectures given in the Medical Centre, Bad Ragaz

Bohannon RW, Andrews AW (1987) Relative strength of seven upper extremity muscle groups in hemiparetic stroke patients. J Neuro Rehabil 1 (4): 161–165

Brodal A (1973) Self-observations and neuro-anatomical considerations after a stroke. Brain 96: 675–694

Bromley J (1976) Tetraplegia and paraplegia, a guide for physiotherapists. Churchill Livingstone, Edinburgh

Brooks VB (1986) The neural basis of motor control. Oxford University Press

Brunstrom S (1970) Movement therapy in hemiplegia: a neurophysiological approach. Harper and Row, New York

Caix M, Outrequin G, Descottes B, Kalfon M, Pouget X (1984) The muscles of the abdominal wall: a new functional approach with anatomo-clinical deductions. Anat Clin 6: 109–116

Campbell EJM, Green JH (1953) The expiratory function of the abdominal muscle in man. an electromyographical study. J Physiol (Lond) 120: 409–418

Campbell EJM, Green JH (1955) The behaviour of the abdominal muscles and the intra-abdominal pressure during quiet breathing and increased pulmonary ventilation. A study in man. J Physiol (Lond) 127: 423–426

Charness A (1986) Stroke/headinjury. Rehabilitation institute of Chicago procedure manual. Aspen, Rockville

Davies PM (1985) Steps to follow. A guide to the treatment of adult hemiplegia. Springer, Berlin Heidelberg New York

De Troyer A (1983) Mechanical action of the abdominal muscles. Bull Eur Physiopathol Respir 19: 575–581

270   References

De Troyer A, De Beyl DZ, Thirton M (1981) Function of the respiratory muscles in acute hemiplegia. Am Rev Respir Dis 123: 631-632

Dettmann MA, Linder MT, Sepic SB (1987) Relationship among walking performance, postural stability, and functional assessment of the hemiplegic patient. Am J Phys Med 66 (2): 77-90

Diamond N (1970) Tap root manuscript. Universal City Records

Donisch FW, Basmajian JV (1972) Electromyography of deep muscles in man. Am J Anat 153: 25-36

Dvorak J, Dvorak V (1983) Manual medicine, diagnostic. Thieme, Stuttgart

Flint MM, Gudgell J (1965) Electromyographic study of abdominal muscular activity during exercise. Am J Phys Med 36: 29-37

Fluck DC (1966) Chest movements in hemiplegia. Clin Sci 31: 383-388

Fugl-Meyer AR, Griemby G (1984) Respiration in tetraplegia and in hemiplegia: a review. Int Rehabil Med 6: 186-190

Fugl-Meyer AR, Linderholm H, Wilson AF (1983) Restrictive ventilatory dysfunction in stroke: its relation to locomotor function. Scand J Rehabil Med [Suppl 9]: 118-124

Gelb M (1987) Body learning: an introduction to the Alexander technique. Aurum, London

Grieve GP (1979) Mobilisation of the spine, 3rd edn. Churchill Livingstone, Edinburgh

Grieve GP (1981) Common vertebral joint problems. Churchill Livingstone, Edinburgh

Grieve GP (ed) (1986) Modern manual therapy of the vertebral column. Churchill Livingstone, Edingburgh

Haas A, Rusk HA, Pelosof H, Adam JR (1967) Respiratory function in hemiplegic patients. Arch Phys Med Rehabil (April): 174-179

Hellebrandt FA (1938) Standing as a geotropic reflex. The mechanism of the asynchronous rotation of motor units. Am J Physiol 121: 471-474

Hellebrandt FA, Braun GL (1939) The influence of sex and age in the postural sway of man. Am J Physiol Anthropol 24: 347-360

Hellebrandt FA, Tepper RH, Braun GL, Elliott MC (1938) The location of the cardinal anatomical orientation plane passing through the center of weight in young adult women. Am J Physiol 121: 465-470

Hellebrandt FA, Brogdon E, Tepper RH (1940) Posture and its cost. Am J Physiol 129: 773-781

Hockermann S, Dickstein R, Pinar T (1984) Platform training and postural stability in hemiplegia. Arch Phys Med Rehabil 65: 588-592

Kesselring J (1989) Theoretische Grundlagen der Sensomotorik zum Verständnis der Therapie ihrer Störungen. Lecture in Postgraduate Study Center Hermitage, Bad Ragaz

Klein-Vogelbach S (1963) Die Stabilisation der Körpermitte und die aktive Widerlagerbildung als Ausgangspunkt einer Bewegungserziehung (unter besonderer Berücksichtigung der Probleme des Hemiplegikers). Krankengymnastik 5: 1-9 (Offprint)

Klein-Vogelbach S (1990) Ballgymnastik zur funktionellen Bewegungslehre. Analysen und Rezepte, 3rd edn. Springer, Berlin Heidelberg New York (Rehabilitation und Prävention, vol 1)

Klein-Vogelbach S (1986) Therapeutische Übungen zur funktionellen Bewegungslehre. Analysen und Rezepte, 2nd edn. Springer, Berlin Heidelberg New York (Rehabilitation und Prävention, vol 4)

Klein-Vogelbach S (1987) Functional kinetics. Lecture for the 3rd IBITAH-meeting in the Postgraduate Study Centre Hermitage, Bad Ragaz

Knott M, Voss DE (1960) Proprioceptive neuromuscular facilitation. Harper, New York

Knuttson E (1981) Gait control in hemiparesis. Scand J Rehabil Med 13: 101-108

Knuttson E, Richards C (1979) Different types of disturbed motor control in gait of hemiplegic patients. Brain 102: 405-430

Kolb LC, Kleyntyens F (1937) A clinical study of the respiratory movements in hemiplegia. Brain 60: 259-274

Korczyn AD, Leibowitz U, Bendermann J (1969a) Involvement of the diaphragm in hemiplegia. Neurology 19: 97-100

Korczyn AD, Hermann G, Don R (1969b) Diaphragmatic involvement in hemiplegia and hemiparesis. J Neurol Neurosurg Psychiat 32: 588-590

Kottke FJ (1975a) Reflex patterns initiated by the secondary sensory fiber endings of muscle spindels: a proposal. Arch Phys Med Rehabil 56: 1-7

Kottke FJ (1975b) Neurophysiologic therapy for stroke. In: Licht S (ed) Stroke and its rehabilitation. Licht, New Haven, pp 256-324

Kottke FJ, Halpern D, Easton JKM, Ozel AT, Burrill CAV (1978) The training of coordination. Arch Phys Med Rehabil 59: 567-572

Kottke FJ (ed) (1982a) The neurophysiology of motor function. Saunders, Philadelphia, pp 218-252 (Krusen's handbook of physical medicine and rehabilitation)

Kottke FJ (ed) (1982b) Therapeutic exercise to develop neuromuscular coordination. Saunders, Philadelphia, pp 403-426 (Krusen's handbook of physical medicine and rehabilitation)

Luce MY, Bruce H, Culver MD (1982) Respiratory muscle function in health and disease. Chest 81: 82-90

Mahoney FI, Barthel DW (1965) Functional evaluation: the Barthel index. Maryland State Med J (February): 61-65

Maitland GD (1986) Vertebral manipulation. Butterworths, London

Middendorf J (1987) Der erfahrbare Atem. Junfermann, Paderborn

Mohr JD (1984-1987) Lectures given during courses on the assessment and treatment of adult patients with hemiplegia: Post Graduate Study Centre Hermitage, Bad Ragaz

Montgomery J (1987) Assessment and treatment of locomotor deficits. In: Duncan PW, Badke MB (eds) Stroke rehabilitation: the recovery of motor control. Year Book Medical, Chicago

Murphy J, Koepke GD, Smith EM, Dickinson AA (1959) Sequence of action of the diaphragm and intercostal muscles during respiration. II: Expiration. Arch Phys Med 40: 337-342

Murray PM, Drought AB, Kory RC (1964) Walking patterns in normal men. Bone Joint Surg 46: 335-345

Murray PM, Seireg AA, Sepic SB (1975) Normal postural stability and steadiness: quantitative assessment. Bone Joint Surg 57: 510-516

Okamoto T (1973) Electromyographic study of the learning process of walking in 1- and 2 year-old infants. Medicine and Sport 8 (Biomechanics III): 328-333

Olney SJ, Monga TN, Costigan PC (1986) Mechanical energy of walking of stroke patients. Arch Phys Med Rehabil 67: 92-98

Pauly JE, Steele RW (1966) Electromyographic analysis of back exercises for paraplegic patients. Arch Phys Med 47: 730-736

Perkins WH, Kent RD (1986) Textbook of functional anatomy of speach, language and hearing. Taylor and Francis, London

Perry J (1969) The mechanics of walking in hemiplegia. Clin Orthop 63: 23-31

Platzer W (1984) Bewegungsapparat. Thieme, Stuttgart, p 84 (Taschenbuch der Anatomie, vol 1)

Raibert MH, Sutherland IE (1983) Maschinen zu Fuss. Spektrum der Wissenschaft 3: 30-40

Rolf HFG, Bressel G, Holland B, Rodatz U (1973) Physiotherapie bei querschnittgelähmten Patienten. Kohlhammer, Stuttgart

Saunders M, Inman VT, Eberhart HD (1953) The major determinants in normal and pathological gait. Bone Joint Surg 35: 543-557

Schultz AB (1982) Low back pain. Biomechanics of the spine. Proceedings of the international symposium organised by the back pain association, held in London, October

Schultz AB, Benson DR, Hirsch C (1974) Force-deformation properties of human ribs. Biomechanics 7: 303-309

Sharp JT (1980) Respiratory muscles: a review of old and newer concepts. Lung 157: 185-199

Sherrington C (1947) The integrative action of the nervous system, 2nd edn. Yale University Press, New Haven

Spaltenholz W (1901) Handbuch der Anatomie des Menschen. Hirzel, Stuttgart, p 277

Steindler A (1955) Kinesiology of the human body under normal and pathological conditions. Thomas, Springfield

Truswell AS (1986) ABC of nutrition. Br Med J, London

Wade T, Langton Hewer R (1987) Functional abilities after stroke: measurement, natural history and prognosis. J Neurol Neurosurg Psychiat 50: 177–182

Williams PL, Warwick R (1980) Gray's anatomy, 36th edn. Churchill Linvingstone, Edinburgh

Winter DA (1983) Energy generation and absorption at the ankle and knee during fast, natural and slow cadences. Clin Orthop 175: 147–154

Wright S (1945) Applied physiology. Oxford University Press, Oxford

Subject Index

S. Klein-Vogelbach, Bottmingen, Switzerland

Functional Kinetics

Observing, Analyzing,
and Teaching Human Movement

Tranlated from the German by G. Whitehouse

1990. XIV, 337 pp. 329 figs. 1 tab. ISBN 3-540-15350-0

Susanne Klein-Vogelbach's acclaimed textbook describing her concept of functional kinetics is now available in English! The well-known physiotherapist has once again revised the material to improve the presentation of her theory concerning the systematic observation and analysis of human movement. The direct observation of movement is an excellent foundation on which to build successful therapeutic programs. The ideas outlined in this book are basic to physical therapy and rehabilitation and should be familiar to every active therapist.

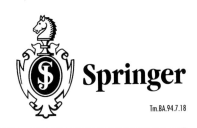

Springer

Preisänderungen vorbehalten

Tm.BA.94.7.18

P. M. Davies, Bad Ragaz

Steps to Follow

A Guide to the Treatment of Adult Hemiplegia

Based on the Concept of K. and B. Bobath

With a Foreword by W. M. Zinn

1984 XXIII, 300 pp. 326 figs. in 492 sep illus. ISBN 3-540-13436-0

The Optimal rehabilitation of the stroke patient requires both time and skillful handling on the part of the therapist. Well-informed relatives can help considerably.

Pat Davies provides a clear guide to the treatment which she has developed during many years of experience as a physiotherapist and a teacher. Based on the concept of Karel and Bertie Bobath, her approach to the rehabilitation of hemiplegic patients stresses the need to equip the patient for a full life, rather than setting arbitary goals for functioning in the hospital or a sheltered environment.

In this book activities are described for preventing and correcting abnormal movement patterns, shoulder problems and facial difficulties. Ways to regain functional walking, balance reactions and many other normal movement sequences are explained and demonstrated with over four hundred photographs of actual patients.

For doctors, physiotherapists, occupational therapists and nurses who work with hemiplegic patients, the book fills a gap in the literature. Their relatives and friends will also be better able to understand the problems they encounter, and find many ideas as to how these can be dealt with.

Preisänderungen vorbehalten

Springer

Tm.BA.94.7.18